AF574512

LYMPHATIC DRAINAGE OF THE SKIN AND BREAST

LYMPHATIC DRAINAGE OF THE SKIN AND BREAST

Locating the Sentinel Nodes

Roger F. Uren
Missenden Medical Centre, Sydney, Australia

John F. Thompson
Royal Prince Alfred Hospital, Sydney, Australia

and

Robert B. Howman-Giles
Missenden Medical Centre, Sydney, Australia

harwood academic publishers
Australia • Canada • China • France • Germany • India • Japan • Luxembourg
Malaysia • The Netherlands • Russia • Singapore • Switzerland

Amsteldijk 166
1st Floor
1079 LH Amsterdam
The Netherlands

British Library Cataloguing in Publication Data

A catalogue record for this book is available from the British Library.

ISBN 90-5702-410-1

Cover illustration: Lyn E. McKenzie

This book is dedicated firstly to my loving wife Maureen and two lovely daughters Katherine and Alexandra. Having a happy peaceful home-life makes any man's work-life easy. Secondly I dedicate this work to my late dear friend Bill Kaplan who first taught me the method of lymphoscintigraphy, and finally I thank John Morris for convincing me to adopt nuclear medicine as my specialty as I have enjoyed a most rewarding academic career in its practice over the last 25 years.

ROGER F. UREN

CONTENTS

PREFACE

Lymphatic mapping, after a very long history, has recently become a subject of great clinical relevance and importance with the development of the sentinel node biopsy technique. It is thus on the cusp of a new and exciting era. The sentinel node concept is creating great interest in surgical oncology as it offers the prospect of accurately staging whole node fields for the presence of metastatic disease by removing and carefully examining only one or two sentinel nodes. This approach is likely to become the standard of care in patients with melanoma when appropriate clinical trials have been completed and is likely to assume a similar role in breast cancer patients. As well, the technique is already being successfully applied to vulval and penile cancer and early studies suggest a possible role in uterine cancer, bowel cancer, and a range of other malignancies which metastasize via the lymphatic system to regional lymph nodes.

This book describes methods which will achieve accurate lymphatic mapping of the skin and breast to ensure confident sentinel node identification in patients with melanoma and breast cancer. All of the lymphoscintigraphy studies were performed at Nuclear Medicine and Diagnostic Ultrasound, Misenden Medical Centre, Camperdown, Australia. The melanoma patients were referred from the Sydney Melanoma Unit, Royal Prince Alfred Hospital, Camperdown and the breast cancer patients were referred by surgeons at BreastScreen NSW.

Central to the successful application of these lymphatic mapping techniques using radiocolloids is a thorough understanding of the way the lymphatic system handles radiocolloids and those features of radiocolloids which are important to achieve accurate and clear mapping. Likewise, correct scanning procedures during cutaneous and breast lymphoscintigraphy require a complete knowledge of the lymphatic drainage pathways possible from each site and an imaging protocol which includes all of them. The technique of marking the location of sentinel nodes during lymphoscintigraphy and the surgical method of harvesting the nodes after blue dye injection, combined with the use of a gamma detection probe during surgery, are also critically important to the successful completion of any sentinel node biopsy procedure.

This book provides a comprehensive description of all of these important aspects of lymphatic mapping and sentinel node biopsy. Particular emphasis is placed on the physiological interaction of radiocolloids with the lymphatic system. This discussion leads directly to a description of the ideal characteristics of radiocolloids for lymphatic mapping. The choice of an appropriate radiocolloid is a vital first step in achieving accurate results in both lymphoscintigraphy and sentinel node biopsy. If the radiocolloid chosen does not accurately map the lymphatic system, it is inevitable that sentinel nodes will be missed and the whole rationale for this surgical approach to staging and treatment will be negated. Scanning protocols required in different parts of the body are described, based on knowledge obtained during more than 2000 studies of the lymphatic drainage of the skin in melanoma patients and over 150 studies in patients with breast cancer. A detailed description of the technique of lymphoscintigraphy is included for both melanoma and breast cancer patients. Unusual drainage patterns which can occur on cutaneous lymphoscintigraphy are emphasized, so that the scanning protocol can be adjusted in each melanoma patient to ensure that such unusual drainage is not missed and that all potential sentinel nodes are thus located for biopsy.

The importance and methods of accurately marking the location of the sentinel nodes during lymphoscintigraphy are described in detail. Surgical technique for sentinel node biopsy is described, and the complimentry roles of blue dye injection and intra-operative use of a gamma detection probe are discussed. The potentially serious pitfalls of using a gamma detection probe alone for sentinel node biopsy, without preoperative lymphoscintigraphy, are also considered.

We hope that nuclear medicine physicians and surgical oncologists will find the book helpful when they come to apply the sentinel node biopsy technique to their patients with melanoma and breast cancer. The new insights into lymphatic anatomy and physiology will also be of interest to anatomists, physiologists and those involved in the care of patients with disorders of the lymphatic system, particularly lymphoedema.

Whenever possible, illustrations have been used to highlight the variability of lymphatic drainage which can be seen in different patients. Many of the figures were produced using Arcview®[1], a geographic information system software package which has allowed the distribution of primary melanoma sites to be mapped out on a normalised body outline. We have also included examples of lymphoscintigrams whenever possible to illustrate the unusual lymphatic pathways which can be seen in individual patients.

Finally we would like to make a plea to all colleagues who are performing or planning to perform sentinel node biopsy procedures. The aim of the sentinel

---

[1] Arcview® GIS by Environmental Systems Research Institute, Inc., Redlands, California 92373, USA.

node biopsy procedure is not to remove a 'hot' node or a 'blue' node, rather it is to accurately map the physiology of lymphatic drainage from the site of the primary tumour and to remove the draining sentinel node or nodes. Non-physiologic interventions such as large volume injections of large colloid particles may lead to a high success rate in finding and removing 'hot' nodes in draining node fields but do not necessarily equate to a sucessful sentinel node biopsy.

FOREWORD

Less than a decade since my original description of intraoperative lymphatic mapping and sentinel lymphadenectomy before the Society of Surgical Oncology, this procedure has been widely adopted. Many investigators have confirmed that the tumor status of the sentinel node (the first draining lymph node on the direct drainage pathway from the primary tumor site) reflects the tumor status of the entire nodal basin. Intraoperative lymphatic mapping and sentinel lymphadenectomy can spare 70–80% of melanoma and breast cancer patients with negative sentinel nodes the trauma of radical lymphadenectomy. However, the technique is technically challenging and places new emphasis on dynamic and accurate cutaneous lymphoscintography to identify the nodal basin at risk and the true sentinel node in that basin. Drs. Uren, Howman-Giles, and Thompson have described and improved the technique that now appears likely to revolutionize the management of melanoma, breast cancer, and many other solid neoplasms that metastasize through the lymphatics.

This is the first comprehensive text to detail the methodology of lymphoscintigraphy of the skin and breast and the surgical techniques of lymphatic mapping and sentinel lymphadenectomy. The authors have the largest experience in the world with these techniques using the huge patient database of the Sydney Melanoma Unit. This monograph represents a careful analysis of this experience based on 1600 cases of melanoma and more than 100 cases of breast cancer. It should be required reading for any physician who treats melanoma or breast cancer because it provides a level of understanding about the anatomy and physiology of the lymphatic system not otherwise available. The book is complete in content and references. Important pitfalls and possible errors are outlined in a straightforward 'how to do it' approach. One of the many strengths of the book is its clear delineation of the complexity and frequency of ectopic drainage patterns in melanoma and breast cancer. Ectopic lymph nodes are much more common than previously realized, and their identification is essential for accurate lymphatic mapping and sentinel lymphadenectomy.

The field of oncology owes a debt of gratitude to Drs. Uren, Howman-Giles, and Thompson for this important monograph, which will be a welcome addition to the library of every surgeon or nuclear medicine physician who cares for patients with melanoma or breast cancer. I predict that this will be the first of many editions updating this important and rapidly evolving field.

DONALD L. MORTON, M.D.
John Wayne Cancer Institute
Santa Monica, California

ACKNOWLEDGEMENTS

We would like to acknowledge the superb work of all the technologists working in nuclear medicine at the Missenden Medical Centre over the past 14 years who have performed the high-quality lymphoscintigrams illustrated in this book. These technologists include Ian Dyer, Sally Raymond, Kim Ioannou, Tracey Smith, Katrina Hoch, Nicholas Trpezanovski and Rhodora Paglinawan. We would like to thank Dr John Roberts and Dr Elizabeth Bernard for their help in supervising some of the lymphoscintigraphy studies used in this series. We would also like to thank all of the surgeons at the Sydney Melanoma Unit including William McCarthy, Michael Quinn, Christopher O'Brien and Gerald Milton, and the surgeons of BreastScreen NSW including Stuart Renwick, David Gillett, George Ramsey-Stewart and Fred Niesche whose encouragement and referrals led to such a large experience being obtained by us over this period. Great assistance in the work was provided by others at the Sydney Melanoma Unit including Helen Shaw, Carla Bosch, Elizabeth Scahill, Lynda Hussein and Gordana Vijuk. Thanks also to the audio-visual department at the Royal Prince Alfred Hospital for their help in preparing the illustrations and to Robert Haynes for his exceptional medical illustration skills.

Chapter 1

LYMPHATICS

1.1 EMBRYOLOGICAL DEVELOPMENT

Although blood vessels begin to develop at about 3 weeks gestation, there are no lymphatics in the early stages of human embryonic development. The primitive lymphatic system can first be identified as pools of fluid within the tissues of the developing embryo at about 5 weeks gestation. As the pressure in the blood vessels increases and partially overcomes the plasma protein osmotic pressure, there begins a slow leakage of fluid and protein into the tissues around the blood vessels. If this fluid was allowed to accumulate without control, interstitial tissue pressures would increase, causing impairment of protein transport and cell function.[1] Toxicity from the products of cell metabolism and cell degradation would also interfere with normal cell function. This build-up of fluid in the interstitial space appears to be the stimulus for development of the lymphatic system.

In simple terms the lymphatic system develops in most tissues to act as the drainage system for metabolic debris, fluid and leaked plasma protein. Once the lymphatic capillaries begin appearing during foetal growth they increase in numbers very rapidly. Sabin showed that in the pig embryo when the crown rump length is about 4 cm, primary lymph sacs form from the venous endothelium at the junction point of the cardinal and subclavian veins on each side at the base of the neck.[2] Similar lymph sacs form over the iliac crest and from these points the lymphatic capillaries of the skin spread rapidly to cover the entire body. Also in the pig embryo the thoracic duct and collecting vessels with functioning valves are able to be identified by the time the crown-rump length is 10 cm.[3]

Lymphatic capillaries develop in a manner which is similar to the development of blood vessels. Mesenchymal cells form cords which then cavitate, after which endothelial cells arrange themselves around the cavities. The lymphatic cavities fuse to form channels which then extend by budding off new channels or fusing in turn with other channels. The major lymphatic channels tend to follow the course of the main veins. The anastomosis of several lymphatic channels forms a series of primary lymph sacs in the foetus. These consist of two jugular lymph sacs, two iliac lymph sacs, a single retroperitoneal lymph sac and the cysterna chyli sac. Finally, the thoracic duct appears on the left and the right lymphatic duct on the right. The lymphatic capillaries and other lymphatic vessels develop before the lymph nodes, though the appearance and growth of the nodes rapidly follows the vessels.

An ability to form lymphatic vessels continues into adult life, so that transplanted tissues including skin will, after a brief period, develop lymph channels which reconnect with the native lymph vessels to provide lymph drainage from the transplanted tissue.[4] These new channels can be demonstrated by lymphoscintigraphy.

Some tissues have no internal lymphatic system and develop an alternative drainage mechanism. The most important of these is the brain, where the lymphatic pools enlarge and coalesce to form a large fluid reservoir — the cerebrospinal fluid space. The skin and breast, however, like most body tissues, develop an extensive system of lymphatic capillaries to act as their drainage system.

1.2 ANATOMY

1.2.1 Lymphatic Vessels

1.2.1.1 *Pre-lymphatics (terminal lymphatics)*

Lymphatic vessels in the skin begin as microtubular pre-lymphatics (also known as terminal lymphatics) in the dermal papillae just below the epidermis.[5] These microtubules appear to be connected to similar irregular microtubules in the region of the basal cells of the epidermis itself. The microtubular pre-lymphatics have endothelial cells in a flat cylindrical configuration which are only loosely attached to each other. There are quite large gaps between cells, and there is almost no protein polysaccharide basement membrane. These gaps at the intercellular junctions can measure up to 2000 to 3000 nanometres in some circumstances and even where the cells are held together at ‘maculae adherentes’ there remain gaps of 10 to 25 nanometres.[6] Occasionally the cells fuse together at zones called ‘maculae occludentes’ and at these points there is no gap. The endothelial cells lining lymphatic capillaries are markedly effaced over the cylindrical shape of the capillary and though they measure 2000–4000 nanometres in thickness across the part of the cell containing the nucleus, they may measure less than 100 nanometres at the point where they meet adjacent endothelial cells.

Lymphatic endothelial cells have many small invaginations on both their luminal and connective tissue surfaces. These are much more common than is found with endothelial cells in blood capillaries. Such invaginations, called caveolae, are found in any cell type which performs pinocytosis (Figure 1.1). They are about 75 nanometres in diameter. Lymphatic endothelial cells also have the usual intracytoplasmic organelles such as the Golgi complex, centrioles, rough endoplasmic reticulum (ER), free ribosomes and mitochondria.[7] The Golgi complex and centrioles in the cell tend to be clustered around the nucleus and are less developed than in endothelial cells lining blood vessels. The rough ER, which is sparse and also poorly developed, is scattered throughout the cytoplasm along with the ribosomes. This paucity of rough ER is indicative of a low level of protein synthesis in lymphatic endothelial cells. Anchoring filaments

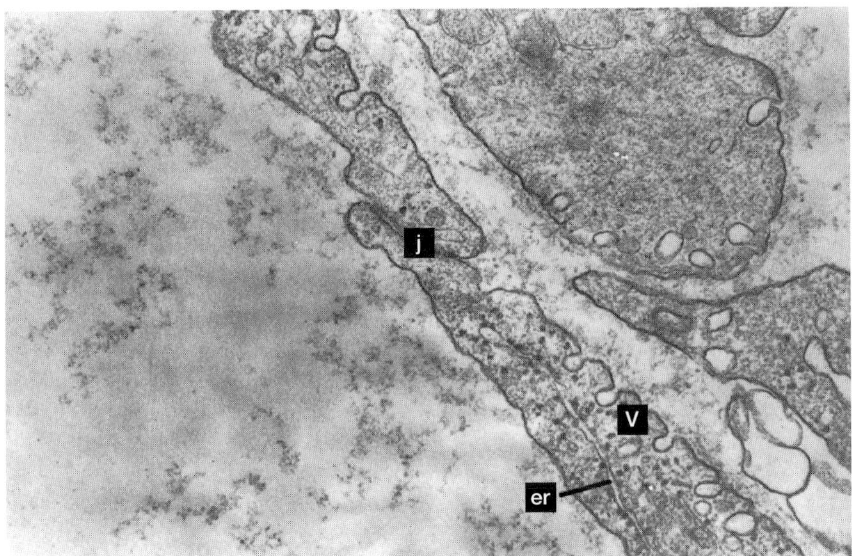

Figure 1.1 Pinocytic vesicles

This EM study at a magnification of ×56,000 shows the junction point (j) of two lymphatic endothelial cells. The cell walls contain many invaginations which form pinocytic vesicles (V) called caveolae. These are about 75 nanometres in diameter. They occur in large numbers in the walls of lymphatic endothelial cells and may play a role in the entry of some colloid particles into the lymphatic capillaries. Some rough endoplasmic reticulum (er) is present in the periphery of the cell. (*Source*: Leak, L.V. (1980) Lymphatic vessels. In *Cardiovascular System, Lymphoreticular and Hematopoietic System*, edited by J.V. Johannessen, pp. 159–183. New York: McGraw-Hill.)

tether the outside of the endothelial cells to the surrounding connective tissue (Figure 1.2). These filaments are elastin microfibrils which are similar in structure to those forming the elastic network of connective tissue.[8]

1.2.1.2 *Lymphatic capillaries*

The micro tubular pre-lymphatic channels coalesce to form lymphatic capillaries of between 20 and 60 micrometres in diameter. Proper lymphatic capillaries are not seen in normal skin above the level of the mid-dermis and are not seen in the dermal papillae. In some disease states, however, lymphatic capillaries appear to open up in these areas and can be clearly seen in the dermal papillae.[9] These

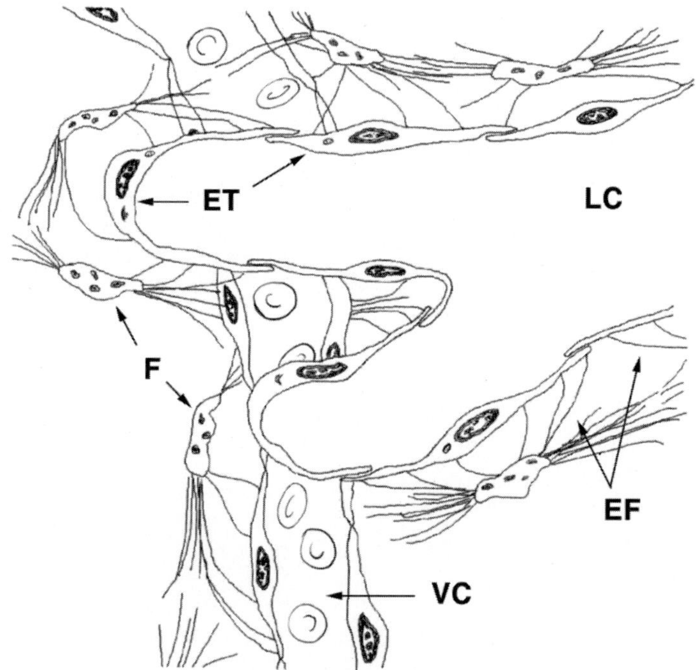

Figure 1.2 Microanatomy of the lymphatic capillaries

The lymphatic capillary endothelial cells (ET) are only loosely associated with each other in the initial lymphatics. The endothelial cells have many elastin fibrils (EF) attached to their outside surfaces which connect the cells to the collagen fibres and fibroblasts (F) in the supporting interstitial matrix. The movement of fluid is from the arterial and venous capillaries (VC) into the interstitial space and from there into the lymphatic capillaries (LC).

larger channels lie in the dermis and can be clearly seen through the skin with the naked eye when injected with a coloured dye. The vessel walls consist of an intima of endothelial cells with occasional muscle cells wrapped around the lymphatic vessel in a spiral fashion. Histologically they have an appearance similar to that of venules. They have smaller gaps at the endothelial junctions, and as they move deeper into the dermis they develop elastic elements and a more complete smooth muscle layer.[1] The junctions of the endothelial cells at this level often overlap (Figure 1.2) to produce valve-like structures which allow fluid, protein and debris to enter the lumen of the lymphatic capillary.[10] Small molecules and water can leave these vessels but large molecules such as proteins cannot, thus the lymph fluid becomes a progressively more concentrated mixture of cells and protein as it passes centrally. There are no intraluminal valves in the pre-lymphatic and lymphatic capillaries and some workers group these two together as the 'initial lymphatics', defining them as that part of the lymphatic system between the beginning of the lymphatic channel and the first intraluminal valve. These initial lymphatics tend to have a tortuous course and anastomose with each other frequently.

1.2.1.3 *Lymphatic collecting vessels*

The lymphatic capillaries join together to form larger collecting vessels (Figure 1.3). The collecting vessels have a 3-layered wall with the endothelial cells forming the inner layer, the smooth muscle cells forming a still incomplete tunica media and the fibroblasts and collagen fibres forming the outer layer. The smooth muscle cells in the tunica media again form an incomplete layer wrapped in a spiral fashion around the endothelial cells so that there are gaps between the muscle cells though these become smaller (Figure 1.4). Valves are found at regular intervals in the collecting vessels spaced about every 2–3 mms along the course of the vessel. Occasionally along the course of the collecting vessels focal dilatation of the vessel occurs where there is pooling of lymph. These lymphatic lakes can sometimes be quite large reaching several millimeters in diameter. On rare occasions a series of lymphatic lakes can be seen along the course of a single lymphatic vessel (Figure 1.5). The collecting lymphatic vessels lie deeper than the initial lymphatics and are much straighter in their course than the initial lymphatics. They tend to run parallel to each other lying in the subcutaneous fat. The collecting vessels have many anastomoses with each other and converge generally towards the veins. They tend to lie superficial to the veins and with the veins they penetrate the deep fascia at the location of major draining node fields such as the groin, the axilla, the popliteal fossa and neck. The most complex part of the lymphatic system draining the skin thus lies superficial to the deep fascia.

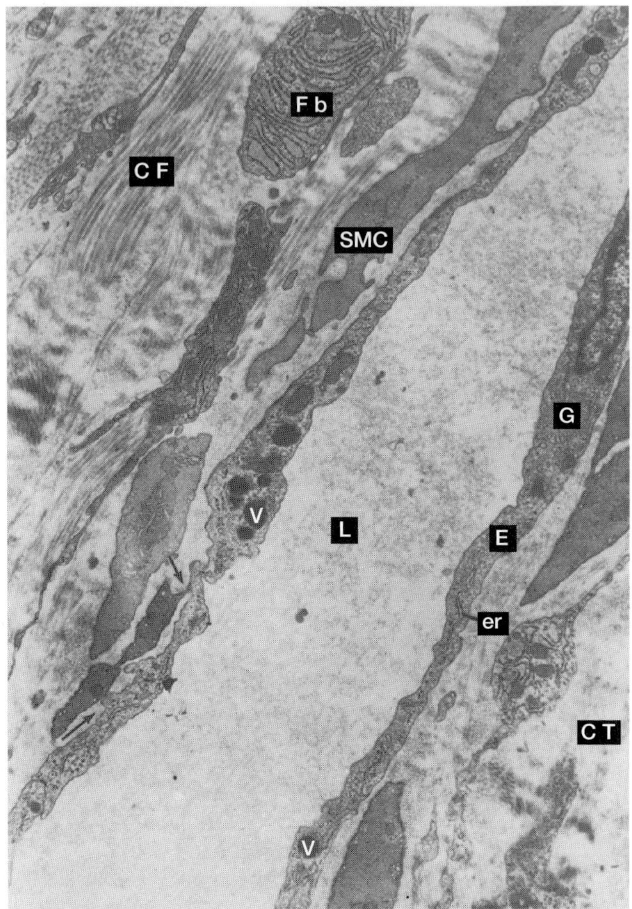

Figure 1.3 A collecting lymph vessel

This EM study at a magnification of ×11,500 shows a collecting lymph vessel. The lumen (L) is lined with endothelial cells (E) which contain vesicles containing electron dense material (V) and the golgi complex (G) is seen near the nucleus. The cells are effaced over the surface of the vessel and contain rough endoplasmic reticulum (er) scattered sparsely about the cell cytoplasm. The smooth muscle cell tunica media layer (SMC) is incomplete and the outside layer of the vessel wall is comprised of fibroblasts (Fb) and collagen fibres (CF) which support the lymphatic vessel in the connective tissue matrix (CT).Arrows point to what appear to be attachments of the smooth muscle cell layer to the outside of the lymphatic endothelial cell wall. (*Source*: Leak, L.V. (1980) Lymphatic vessels. In *Cardiovascular System, Lymphoreticular and Hematopoietic System*, edited by J.V. Johannessen, pp. 159–183. New York: McGraw-Hill.)

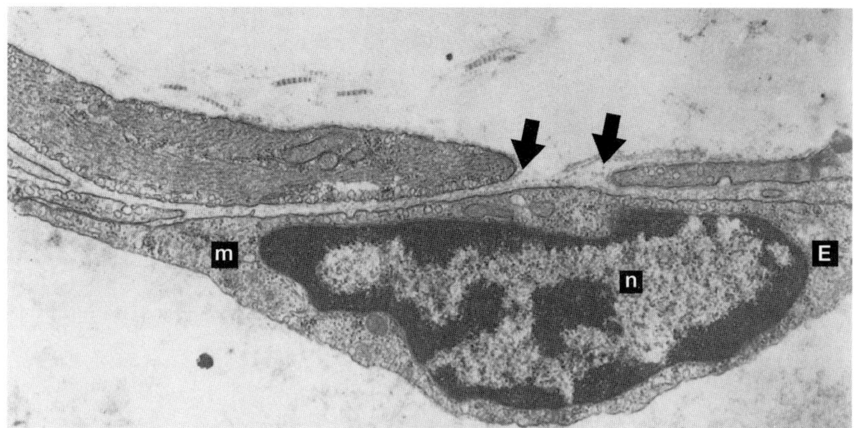

Figure 1.4 The tunica media is incomplete

The smooth muscle cell layer of the lymphatic capillaries and collecting vessels is incomplete with the muscle cells wrapped around the lymph vessel in a spiral fashion. Gaps are thus present between the muscle cells in the tunica media and this EM study at a magnification of 36,000 shows such a gap (arrows). The nucleus (n) is seen in the widest part of the lymphatic endothelial cell (E) and mitochondria (m) are seen characteristically in the perinuclear region of the cell. (*Source*: Leak, L.V. (1980) Lymphatic vessels. In *Cardiovascular System, Lymphoreticular and Hematopoietic System*, edited by J.V. Johannessen, pp. 159–183. New York: McGraw-Hill.)

1.2.1.4 *Major lymphatic trunks*

The lymphatic collecting vessels pass centrally to lymph nodes. Lymphatic fluid may pass through several lymph nodes before eventually reaching the major lymphatic trunks. The major lymph channels from the lower limbs and abdomen form the cisterna chyli in the lumbar region. This is a dilated lymphatic reservoir which is variable in shape. It terminates at about the level of the 1st or 2nd lumbar vertebra where it becomes the thoracic duct. The thoracic duct passes up through the thorax in the prevertebral space to the right of the aorta. It is 2 to 5 mm in diameter and at about the level of the 5th thoracic vertebra it passes to the left and curves up and anteriorly to enter the confluence of the left internal jugular and left subclavian veins.[11] The thoracic duct on the left drains the lower body, left chest and left arm and left side of the head and neck. One or more smaller lymphatic ducts on the right drain the right side of the head and neck, the right arm and the right side of the chest. The thoracic duct and right lymphatic ducts join the venous circulation at about the junction of the internal jugular and subclavian veins. In some patients the internal jugular trunk, inter-

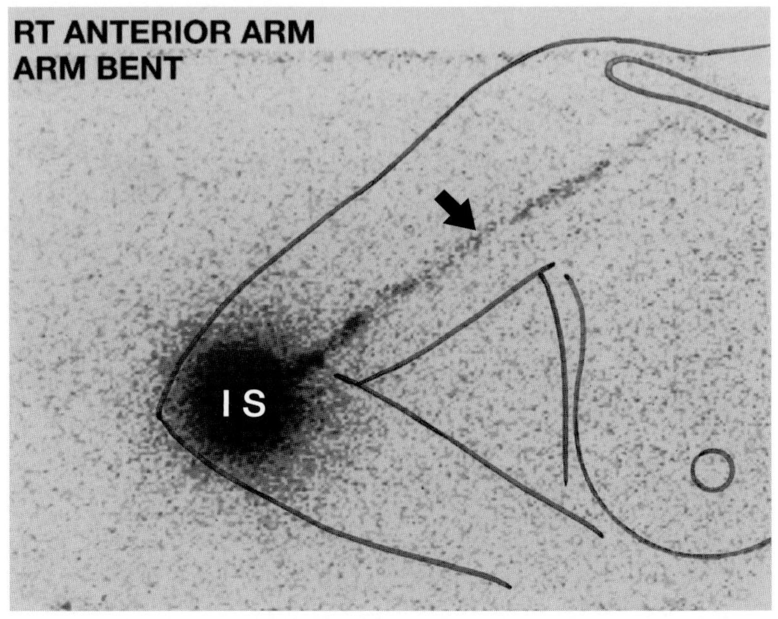

A

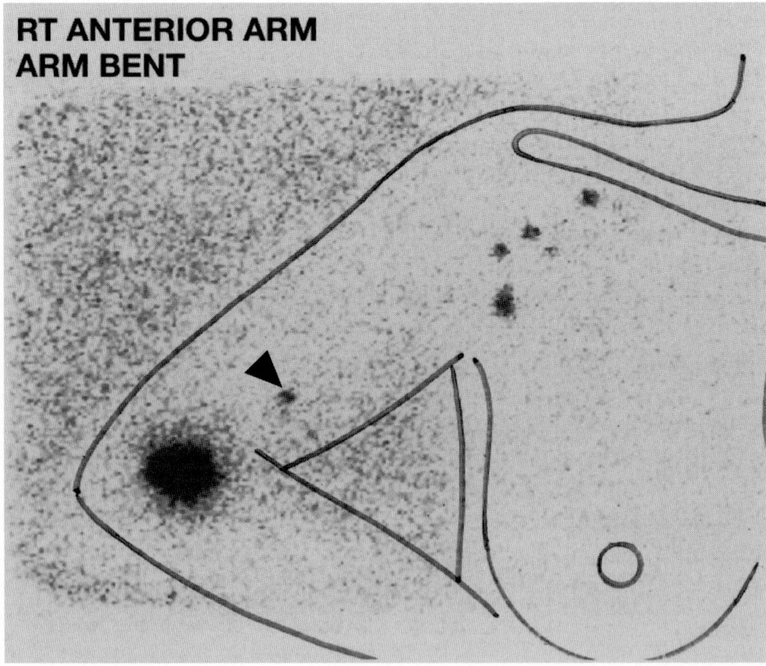

B

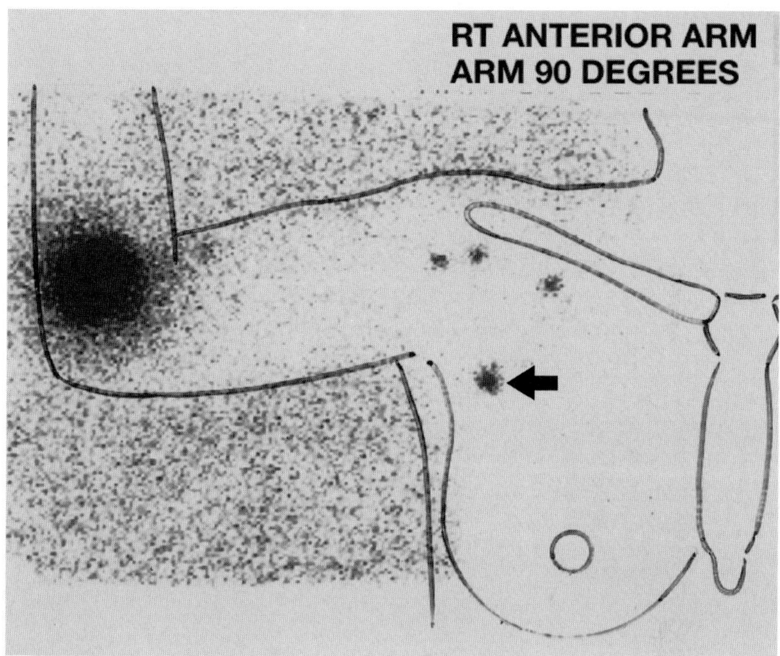

Figure 1.5 Lymphatic lakes

A: In this dynamic phase of lymphoscintigraphy in a patient with a melanoma excision biopsy site (IS) on the lateral right forearm just below the elbow a single dominant channel is seen passing towards the apex of the right axilla (arrow). B: On the delayed scan with the arm down there appears to be an interval node in the arm above the elbow (arrowhead) and several nodes in the right axilla. C: With the arm up the small accumulations of tracer are seen to lie along the course of a lymphatic vessel which traces a curvilinear path to a single sentinel node in the right axilla (arrow). These all proved to be lymphatic lakes when examined at surgery. This appearance is quite unusual, as when present, lymphatic lakes are usually solitary in any one lymphatic vessel.

nal mammary trunk and subclavian trunk join the confluence of the subclavian and internal jugular veins independent of the thoracic duct and right lymphatic duct. These major lymphatic trunks measure 4–6 mm in diameter in man and have a 3-layered wall. They consist of an inner layer of endothelial cells, a complete mid layer of muscle cells with supporting collagen and elastic fibres and an outer layer of fibrous connective tissue, as well as some nerve axons which innervate the muscle cell layer.[7]

1.2.1.5 *Lymphatic valves*

Valves are present in the lumen of the collecting vessels, which lie in the mid to deep dermis (Figure 1.6). The valves ensure that the flow of lymph is mainly unidirectional, though some minor retrograde movement of lymph can be observed in normal lymphatic vessels.[12] The valves are formed of cuspid leaflets joined at the base and sides to form vascular pockets between the valve cusp and the lymphatic capillary wall. The valves are bicuspid and each cusp has two

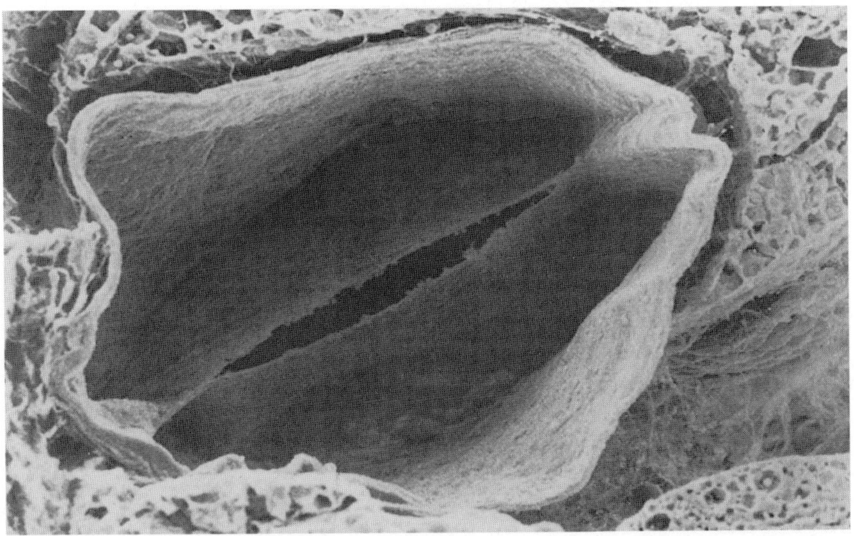

Figure 1.6 Lymphatic valves

This EM study at a magnification of ×400 shows a lymph valve in the thoracic duct. The valve has paired leaflets which interdigitate perfectly with each other to ensure the integrity of the valve when it closes. (*Source*: Leak, L.V. (1980) Lymphatic vessels. In *Cardiovascular System, Lymphoreticular and Hematopoietic System*, edited by J.V. Johannessen, pp. 159–183. New York: McGraw-Hill.)

endothelial walls and a connective tissue core which looks rather like a simple infolding of the lymph vessel wall lining. This, however, is not the case. There are small extensions at the free margin of the valve cusp which interdigitate with the other cusp to facilitate valve closure and there is also a complete basement membrane lining the valvular pocket on the downstream side of the valve.[13] This strengthens the valve and limits retrograde flow of lymph during contraction of the lymphatic pump. The other side of the valve cusp does not have a complete basement membrane, in common with the endothelial lining of lymphatic capillaries generally. The cytoplasm of the endothelial cells which make up the valve also contains numerous filaments which are common in the normal lymphatic endothelial cell. These filaments appear to be actin filaments which have contractile properties[14] and they may thus be able to open the valve to facilitate lymph movement through the lymphatic vessels. Valves occur every 2 to 3 mm along the course of the collecting vessels and Sappey[15] counted 60–80 valves from the fingertip to the axilla. Spontaneous contractions of the lymphatic capillary wall above and below a valve are also timed so that the lymph fluid is propelled centrally.[16] An increase in the intraluminal pressure is associated with increased contractility of smooth muscle elements in the lymphatic wall[17] which also increases central movement of the lymph. The large lymphatic vessels towards the thoracic duct contract spontaneously once every 10 to 15 seconds[18] causing their contents to drain into the venous system.

1.2.2 Lymph Nodes

A lymph node is a discrete structure composed of dense collections of lymphocytes, plasma cells and macrophages surrounded by a capsule of mature collagen. Afferent lymphatic channels enter the cortex of the node through the capsule, draining lymph into the subcapsular sinus (Figure 1.7). The sinuses have many fine reticulin fibres traversing their lumen which trap any particulate matter passing through them. Cortical sinuses arise from the subcapsular sinus and pass towards the medulla of the node where they become known as medullary sinuses. These eventually coalesce to form the efferent lymphatic channels through which lymph leaves the node and passes centrally, eventually to enter the thoracic duct. The subcapsular sinus has only a partial lining of endothelium, as do the cortical sinuses, which means that the cells of the cortex and medulla have direct contact with the lymph fluid contained in the sinuses. Thus the lymphocytes, plasma cells, macrophages and histiocytes can be thought of as partially lining the sinuses. As these sinuses pass towards the medulla, macrophages become the most prominent cells lining their walls.[19] These macrophages are sometimes referred to as sinus histiocytes.

Fibrous trabeculae within a lymph node organise the lymphocytes into cortical follicles and also act as the scaffolding for the subscapular and cortical

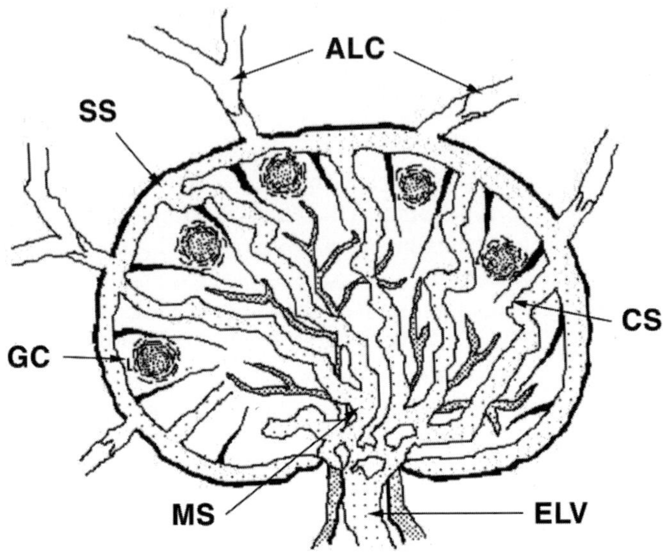

Figure 1.7 Schematic diagram of a lymph node

The afferent lymphatic channels (ALC) pass through the fibrous capsule of the lymph node to enter the subcapsular sinus (SS). These subcapsular sinuses are continuous with the sinuses which pass through the node to become the cortical (CS) and medullary sinuses (MS). Eventually these coalesce to form the efferent lymphatic vessels (ELV) which leave the node generally at the hilum. All of the sinuses contain a fine mesh of reticulin fibres which act as a filter to trap particulate matter. The sinuses are also lined by lymphocytes, histiocytes and macrophages. Germinal centres (GC) are seen scattered throughout the cortex of the node.

sinuses. As already mentioned, these are continuous with the medullary sinuses and eventually with the efferent lymphatics which emerge from the hilum of the lymph node. Lymphoid follicles consist primarily of small B lymphocytes. They have a central zone of proliferating cells called a germinal centre. In this area the lymphocytes are larger and macrophages are also seen. The germinal centres are areas in which significant lymphopoiesis occurs in response to antigenic stimulation. The deepest part of the lymph node cortex, adjacent to the medulla of the node, is called the paracortex and contains sheets of lymphocytes. Specialised blood vessels called post-capillary venules occur in this region of the lymph node and are characterised by a tall endothelial cell lining which is thought to be a special adaptation to allow the movement of large numbers of small lymphocytes across the vessel wall. Most investigators believe that the predominant movement of these small lymphocytes is from the blood to the node[20], and it is thought that the large number of small lymphocytes present in the paracortex come via this mechanism. However, others have proposed that the major movement of the lymphocytes is from the node to the blood.[21] The paracortex has more T lymphocytes, with a 3:1 ratio of T to B lymphocytes, while the medulla contains mostly B lymphocytes and macrophages. The T cells in the paracortex are mainly helper lymphocytes and are important in the induction of B cell responses to antigens which enter the node. When antigens such as radiolabelled colloids enter the node via the afferent lymphatic channels they are first caught in the reticulum mesh of fibres which are present in the sinuses and are then trapped by macrophages, which are concentrated in the sinuses and in the deep cortex.[22] Such macrophages are found especially in the subcapsular sinus and the medullary sinus.[23] Though the situation illustrated schematically in Figure 1.7 is the commonest arrangement, sometimes the major lymph vessels will completely pass through or bypass a node. In this situation the node does not filter the lymph passing along that vessel. Ludwig described 5 different arrangements of afferent and efferent lymphatics in relation to the draining lymph nodes, several of which had at least some of the lymph fluid bypassing the filter function of the node.[24]

With increasing age lymph nodes tend to become smaller, losing some of their lymphoid elements. The number of nodes however does not change. At one time it was thought that lymph nodes could regenerate after surgical removal of a node field had occurred, however this it now not thought to occur.[25]

1.3 PHYSIOLOGY

1.3.1 Major Functions

The major functions of the lymphatic system include the production of small lymphocytes which play a key role in cellular immunity and the production of large lymphocytes which are capable of synthesising antibodies. The lymphatic system also acts as a drainage system to return interstitial fluid and protein to the venous circulation, while the lymph nodes act as filters for debris and infective agents which have gained access to the lymphatic capillaries. In the gut the lymphatic vessels carry absorbed fats to the blood via the thoracic duct, so that metabolism of the fats can commence. The major function of the lymphatic system which is of interest in the present discussion, however, is the movement of interstitial fluid, protein, cell debris and products of cell metabolism via the lymphatic vessels and lymph nodes back to the blood stream from the skin and breast. If these substances were allowed to accumulate in the interstitial space, oedema would rapidly supervene and tissue function and metabolism would be unable to proceed normally.

1.3.2 Lymph Formation

Approximately 90–95% of lymph is formed by capillary filtration as fluid leaks out of capillaries into the interstitial space and is not directly reabsorbed into the venous capillaries (Figure 1.2). The other 5–10% is produced by cells during aerobic metabolism. In a normally active human about 1000 litres of oxygen per day are consumed during the intracellular aerobic metabolism of food. This results in the production of 150–300 ml of water.[26] Fluid, protein, cellular debris and occasional whole cells in the interstitium enter the lymphatic system, initially via the micro-tubular pre-lymphatics. This is the key interface between the interstitial tissues (and the fluid contained therein) and the lymphatic capillary network. The majority of the material which eventually forms the lymphatic fluid enters the system at this interface. The loose connection between cells in the pre-lymphatics allows a free movement of fluid and debris up to 25 nanometres in diameter into the lumen of the pre-lymphatics (Figure 1.8), whilst the larger gaps allow more sizeable molecules and whole cells to enter. Movement in the soft tissues causes tension on the elastin fibrils which attach to the endothelial cells lining the walls of the pre-lymphatic micro-tubule (Figure 1.2). This pulls on the cells and opens up the gaps present between them at this level, thus allowing entry of quite large particles into the lymphatic system.[27] Gaps of 100–500 nanometres are produced in this way (Figure 1.9).[28] Occasionally gaps of 2000–3000 nanometres occur, especially in the presence of inflammation. In the fully formed lymphatic capillary where the endothelial cell junctions are tight, their overlapping structure forms a valve-like mechanism which allows entry of fluid, protein and debris into the lumen. The intraluminal pressure in these micro-tubules and capillaries under basal conditions is usually negative, which further encourages this movement.[29] However, the intraluminal pressure in the larger lymphatic capillaries is positive and has been measured at between 3.9 and 4.5 mmHg in the supine resting human.[30,31] Once the intraluminal pressure rises, the valve mechanism produced by the overlapping endothelial cells closes. Although the structure of the lymphatic capillaries is quite delicate, this overlapping valve mechanism works very efficiently to keep the contents of the lymphatic capillaries inside the lumen. The system maintains its integrity even at high artificial pressures. The very early work of Sappey established that lymphatic capillaries could contain a pressure of up to 80 cm of mercury without rupturing.[32]

Some propose that the osmotic pressure caused by proteins in the lymphatic capillaries is a factor in pulling fluid into the lumen. The weight of evidence, however, suggests that this is not an important mechanism in most circumstances.

Some materials may be transported across the lymphatic endothelial cell and enter the lymphatic lumen by the process of pinocytosis, via the formation of vesicles from the invaginations in the endothelial cell wall which were men-

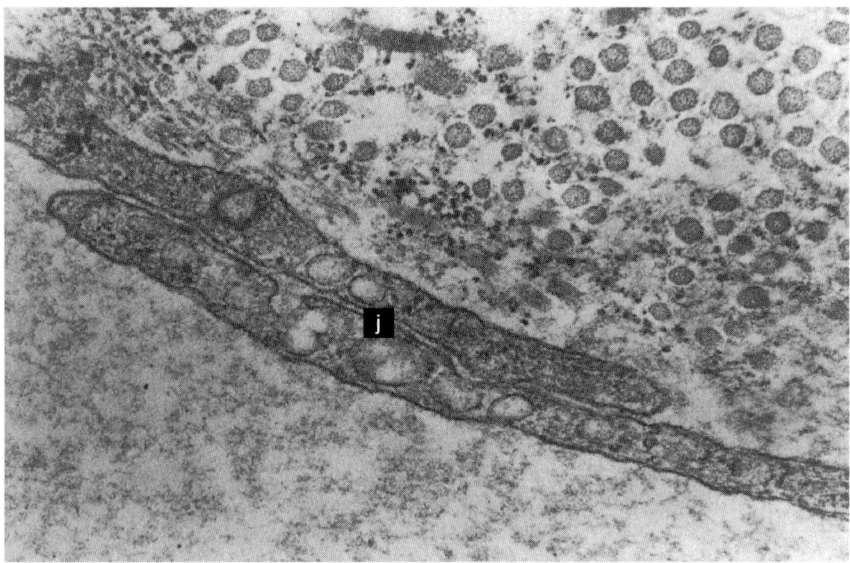

Figure 1.8 The junction between overlapping lymphatic endothelial cells

Lymphatic endothelial cells overlap with each other to form a valve like mechanism which allows fluid into the lumen but when the luminal pressure rises closes to stop fluid leaking out. The gap between the cells where they overlap (j) is 10–25 nanometers which allows particles in this size range ready access to the lumen of the lymphatic capillaries. This EM study at a magnification of ×73,000 shows that the endothelial cells are quite effaced at their point of overlap. (*Source*: Leak, L.V. (1980) Lymphatic vessels. In *Cardiovascular System, Lymphoreticular and Hematopoietic System*, edited by J.V. Johannessen, pp. 159–183. New York: McGraw-Hill.)

tioned earlier (see Figure 1.1).[33, 34] Such pinocytosis has been demonstrated in electron micrographs, where particles have been shown within invaginations of the capillary endothelial plasma membrane and in vesicles in both the peripheral and deeper regions of the cytoplasm.[35] However, these invaginations occur on both sides of the endothelial cell and vesicular movement is not unidirectional within the cell. Movement of material via this mechanism can occur both from the interstitial space to the cell cytoplasm and from the lumen of the lymphatic capillary to the cell cytoplasm. This has been observed following interstitial injection of carbon particles, which have been shown to accumulate in large vacuoles in the cytoplasm of lymphatic endothelial cells (see Figure 1.3). These remain for up to 12 months following interstitial injection. These findings suggest that although pinocytosis may play a role in lymph production, this is

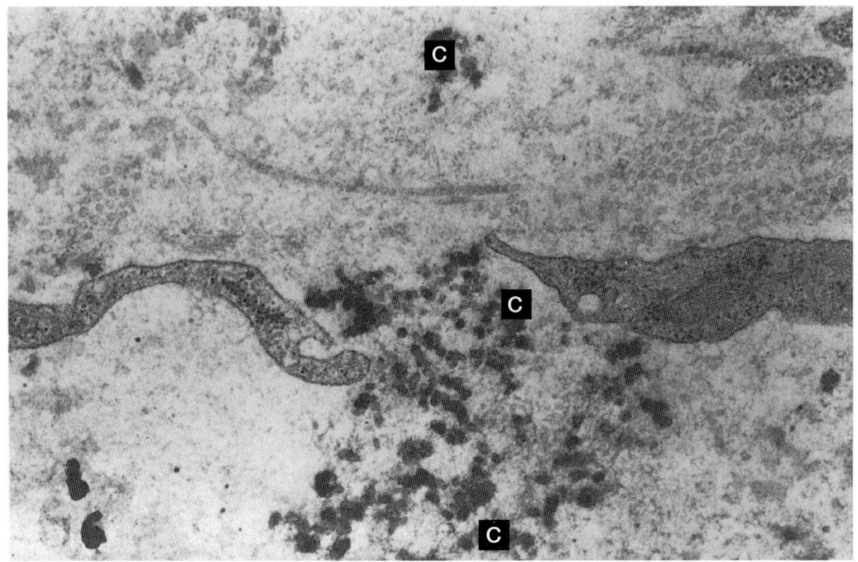

Figure 1.9 Gaps open up between lymphatic endothelial cells

When there is movement of the tissues the elastin fibrils attached to the outside of the lymphatic endothelial cells can pull on the cells and cause wide gaps to open up allowing larger colloidal particles to enter the lymphatic lumen. This EM study at a magnification of ×38,000 shows colloidal carbon particles (C) passing through a gap opened up between lymphatic endothelial cells 24 hours after injection of the colloid. (*Source*: Leak, L.V. (1980) Lymphatic vessels. In *Cardiovascular System, Lymphoreticular and Hematopoietic System*, edited by J.V. Johannessen, pp. 159–183. New York: McGraw-Hill.)

probably a minor part of the process under normal circumstances. Most lymph would appear to enter the lymphatic capillaries via the gaps between endothelial cells and along the intercellular clefts, as described earlier.

1.3.3 Volume of Lymph Production

The volume of lymph fluid produced at any given time is variable and depends on many factors including the ambient temperature and exercise. A normal moving limb has been shown to produce a lymph flow of 0.003 ml/min/100g of tissue.[36] It is estimated that in a normally active human about 2 to 3 litres of lymph fluid re-enters the venous system each day via the thoracic duct and other major lymphatic ducts.[26, 37] An increase in arterial flow such as occurs in association with inflammation will increase the rate of formation of lymph fluid.

Venous occlusion also causes an increase in lymph fluid production, with rapid engorgement of the lymphatic capillaries.[38]

1.3.4 Normal Lymph Flow Rates

Lymph flow is essentially unidirectional from peripheral tissues to the central parts of the body. Lymph eventually re-enters the venous system via the major lymphatic ducts, most via the thoracic duct. Using a 150,000 molecular weight compound, fluorescein isothiocyanate-dextran, injected into the subepidermal layer in the dorsum of the foot, the flow rate in individual 55 micron diameter lymphatic capillaries in humans was measured at 3.1 cm/min.[39] This occurred in the immediate post-injection phase. At the end of the filling period the flow was only 576 microns/min. This dramatic difference was thought to be due to higher interstitial pressure in the initial filling phase. A resting flow rate of 282 microns/min was measured in the tail skin of mice during a constant pressure intradermal injection.[12] The interstitial pressure at the site of the terminal lymphatics affects the uptake of material into the lymphatic capillary but does not appear to alter the net flow velocity.[40] This suggests that lymph flow is determined predominantly by an intrinsic mechanism, possibly the lymphatic pump, plus the sucking action on the thoracic duct created by negative intrathoracic pressure during inspiration. We have found that lymph flow rates in the skin vary systematically with body site and that lymph flow from the breast is generally slower than it is from the skin.[41]

1.3.5 Factors Affecting Lymph Flow

1.3.5.1 *Movement of the tissues*

Movements which induce the passage of material into the lymphatic system include muscle contraction, arterial pulsation, respiration and vibration or twisting of the connective tissue.[42] All of these movements cause traction on the elastin fibrils connecting the endothelial cells in the walls of the lymphatic capillaries to the collagen fibres in the surrounding dermal or mammary connective tissue matrix (Figure 1.2). This traction causes the gaps between the lymphatic endothelial cells to widen, allowing more fluid to enter the lymphatic capillaries.[10]

1.3.5.2 *Tissue compliance and temperature*

The effectiveness of these mechanisms in enhancing the movement of fluid into lymphatics is dependent on the compliance of the tissue concerned. Because the ambient temperature has a significant effect on tissue compliance, a fall in temperature will significantly reduce the movement of fluid and debris into lymphatic vessels. On the other hand movement, exercise, heat and massage will enhance this mechanism and increase lymph flow.[43, 44]

1.3.5.3 *The intrinsic lymphatic pump*

There is good evidence that spontaneous contraction of lymph vessels aids forward motion of the lymph fluid they contain. Using phase analysis it has been shown that the lymph vessel below a valve contracts slightly before the vessel above the valve, thus propelling lymph in a forward direction.[16] Franzeck et al. have shown that such spontaneous contractions in lymphatic capillaries increase significantly in the sitting position compared to the supine position.[30] This intrinsic pump action will propel lymph fluid centrally when the normal muscle pump is inactive during quiet sitting. It has also been noted that the lymphatic capillary pressure increases in the sitting position compared to the supine position (9.9 versus 3.9 mmHg). The stroke volume of the lymphatic pump and the contraction frequency both increase when the lymphatic filling pressure rises to 10 cm H_2O, which may explain the changes observed in the sitting posture.[45] When the flow versus pressure relationship is measured in lymphatic vessels it is found to be non-linear. This non-linearity is due to the lymphatic pump and this can be confirmed by abolishing the lymphatic pump mechanism with verapamil, a calcium channel blocker, after which the flow versus pressure relationship becomes linear.[46] It is thus thought that the lymphatic pump plays a significant role in maintaining lymph flow especially when the body part is inactive.

1.3.5.4 *Gravity*

With the exception of the relatively minor effect on the lymphatics produced by changes in hydrostatic pressure, gravity does not appear to influence lymph flow. LS studies for cutaneous melanoma are usually performed with the patient supine or prone during the dynamic phase, nevertheless there are marked variations in lymph flow depending on the body site being studied. Patients are then upright for 2–2½ hours before delayed scans are performed and new node fields do not appear under the influence of gravity during this period. In fact a much larger area of the trunk drains upwards to the axillary nodes against the pull of gravity than downwards to the groin nodes. Likewise flow can occur up to Level II cervical nodes from primary sites at the base of the neck. In general, however, lymph flow occurs in a central direction regardless of the force of gravity.

1.3.5.5 *Chemical and humoral agents*

The contractile properties of human lymphatics are affected by various chemicals, though there are significant regional variations in the strength of the contractile response to such agents. Contractions are induced by noradrenaline, 5-hydroxytryptamine, prostaglandin F2alpha and U-44069, a thromboxane A2 mimetic. Such contractions are abolished in the presence of phentolamine but are unaffected by propranolol.[47]

1.3.5.6 *Inflammation*

Inflammation in the skin or breast will increase the rate of lymphatic flow due to both an increase in lymph production and an increase in the ambient temperature of the tissues involved. This increases tissue compliance and thus makes any movement in the tissues more effective in increasing lymph flow.

1.3.5.7 *Increased interstitial pressure*

Increased interstitial pressure increases the rate of lymph flow[39] and is also likely to be a factor in inflamed tissue. It has been known for some time that the lymphatic uptake of large particle radiocolloids in lymphoscintigraphy can be improved by injecting larger volumes at each injection site. This forces the larger particles into the lymphatic capillaries by opening up large gaps between the endothelial cells lining the vessel wall. In this way channels and nodes will be visualised in situations where a small volume injectate of the same radiocolloid would not have entered the lymphatic system, resulting in failure of the test.

1.3.5.8 *Venous occlusion*

We have observed a marked increase in lymph flow in patients with venous occlusion, presumably due to a marked increase in lymph production caused by the increased venous pressures. Others have also documented this finding.[38] There is normally no major difference between lymphatic capillary pressure and venous pressure in the leg in the supine position (3.9 versus 6.8 mmHg), but there is a marked difference in the sitting position (9.9 versus 53.3 mmHg).[30] The increased lymph production caused by this pressure differential in the sitting position is counteracted by increased spontaneous contractions of the lymph vessels, as mentioned earlier. Though increased lymph flow is the expected result of venous occlusion, some have found that in patients with chronic venous insufficiency and leg ulcers there is a reduction in lymph flow.[48] This reduced lymphatic drainage may be a factor contributing to the development of ulcers in these patients.

1.3.6 Implications for Preoperative Blue Dye Injection

The importance of these mechanisms in generating and moving lymphatic fluid has major implications for the timing of blue dye injection prior to sentinel node surgery. A cold anaesthetised patient will not demonstrate movement of dye and this will seriously compromise the effectiveness of the technique. The preoperative patient should therefore be kept warm and should be injected with the blue dye while conscious so that a brief period of limb movement or exercise can be undertaken prior to the induction of anaesthesia. This optimises the uptake of the dye and its movement through the lymphatic capillaries. Gentle massage over the injection sites is also an important physiological intervention which increases the movement of injected dye into the lymphatic capillaries and therefore improves the chance of finding a blue stained sentinel node at surgery.

Chapter 2

THE HISTORY OF LYMPHATIC MAPPING

2.1 SOMETHING OTHER THAN BLOOD VESSELS?

Aristotle (384–322 BC), in his work *History of Animals*, used several phrases which suggested that he had observed lymphatic vessels. However, according to Galenic writings it was Herophilus (300 BC) who first noticed lymphatic vessels terminating in glands in the mesentery, and Herasistratus (280 BC) who first described the milky contents of such vessels.[32] Neither recognised these vessels as separate from the blood vessels, with the former believing that they were veins and the latter that they were arteries. Galen mentioned their work only to deny its significance.

2.2 THE FIRST MENTION OF LYMPHATICS

In 1532 Massa described lymphatics in the kidney.[49] The thoracic duct in the horse was discovered by Eustachius in 1563. In 1622 Gasparo Aselli[50], a professor of anatomy and surgery in Pavia, Italy, showed the existence of lymphatic vessels in many different animals including the dog, cat, lamb, cow, pig and horse, and like Herophilus he noticed these vessels joining mesenteric glands.[32] They mistakenly thought that the 'lacteal fluid' then drained to the liver.

Jean Pecquet, of Dieppe, France, in 1649 showed that these vessels passed onwards, to converge at the commencement of the thoracic duct. This confluence he called the cistern or reservoir of the chyle, which later became known as the cisterna chylae. He also accurately described the thoracic duct and the right lymphatic duct, and their entry into the confluence of the internal jugular and subclavian veins on each side.[51]

2.3 INITIAL DENIAL OVERCOME

At about this time both Riolan and Harvey denied the presence of the 'lacteal veins' of Aselli, but subsequent work by Gassendi (1628), Vessling (1634), Folius and Tulpius (1639), Wallee (1641) and Pecquet (1649) confirmed the existence of such vessels.[32] Vessling and Rudbeck showed that these vessels were present in many parts of the body and the systematic study of the lymphatic system was thus commenced. The first mention of the term lymphatic is attributed to Thomas Bartholin in 1653.

2.4 LYMPHATIC VALVES AND OTHER CONCEPTS

In 1665 Olof Rudbeck of Uppsala, with Thomas Bartholin of Copenhagen and others, described valves in the lumen of lymphatic vessels, and Nuck, Hale, Meckel, Haller and Cruickshank showed a wider distribution of such vessels than had previously been thought.[52] William Hunter at his school of anatomy in London stressed the important of the lymphatic system in the process of absorption of fluid from the tissues, and William Hewson, one of his pupils as was William Cruickshank, also contributed with his studies in fish, stating that the superficial and internal lymphatic systems were different.[53] He also suggested that some lymphatic vessels in mammals entered the thoracic duct without traversing a lymph gland. Cruickshank himself produced an important monograph in 1786, *The Anatomy of the Absorbing Vessels of the Human Body*, which contained the most detailed illustrations of the human lymphatics seen up until that time (Figure 2.1).[52] Paolo Mascagni, a professor of anatomy at Siena, Italy, was the first to stress the importance of the origin of the lymphatic vessels in the interstitial fluid, and stated that such vessels did not have any connection with the blood system at the tissue level.[54] He also published an atlas of the lymphatic vessels in man which in detail was a significant advance on that produced by Cruickshank (Figure 2.2). In 1824 Lauth established that each lymphatic vessel had its origin as a network of smaller lymphatics.[55]

2.5 SAPPEY COMMENCES HIS WORK

In 1847 Sappey, a professor of anatomy in Paris, started his extensive research into the lymphatics which culminated in the publication of a large atlas in 1874.[15] His illustrations became classics and were the basis of the general understanding of the cutaneous and mammary lymphatics to the present day (Figure 2.3).

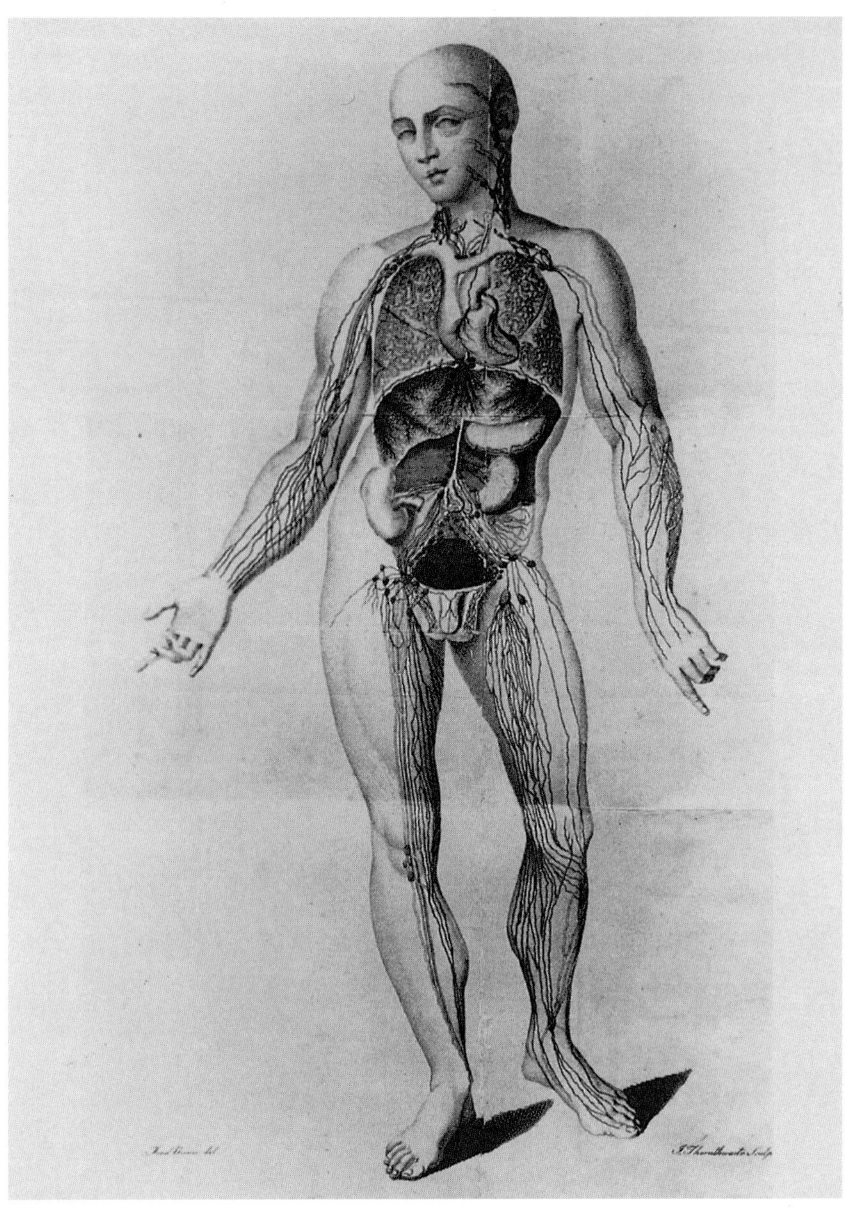

Figure 2.1 Cruikshank's atlas

Cruikshank produced the first detailed atlas of the lymphatics of the human body and his drawings were remarkably accurate.

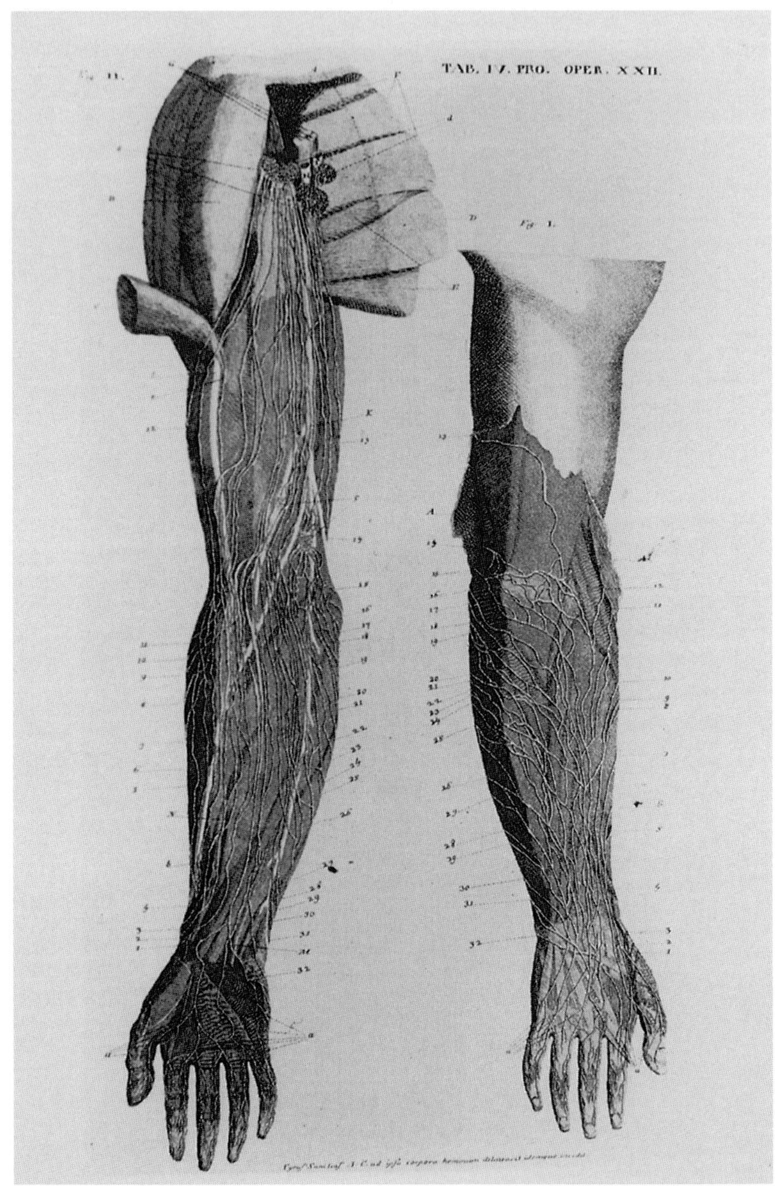

Figure 2.2 Mascagni's atlas

Mascagni improved on the description of the lymphatic vessels and his were the most detailed drawings of the lymphatic channels up to that time.

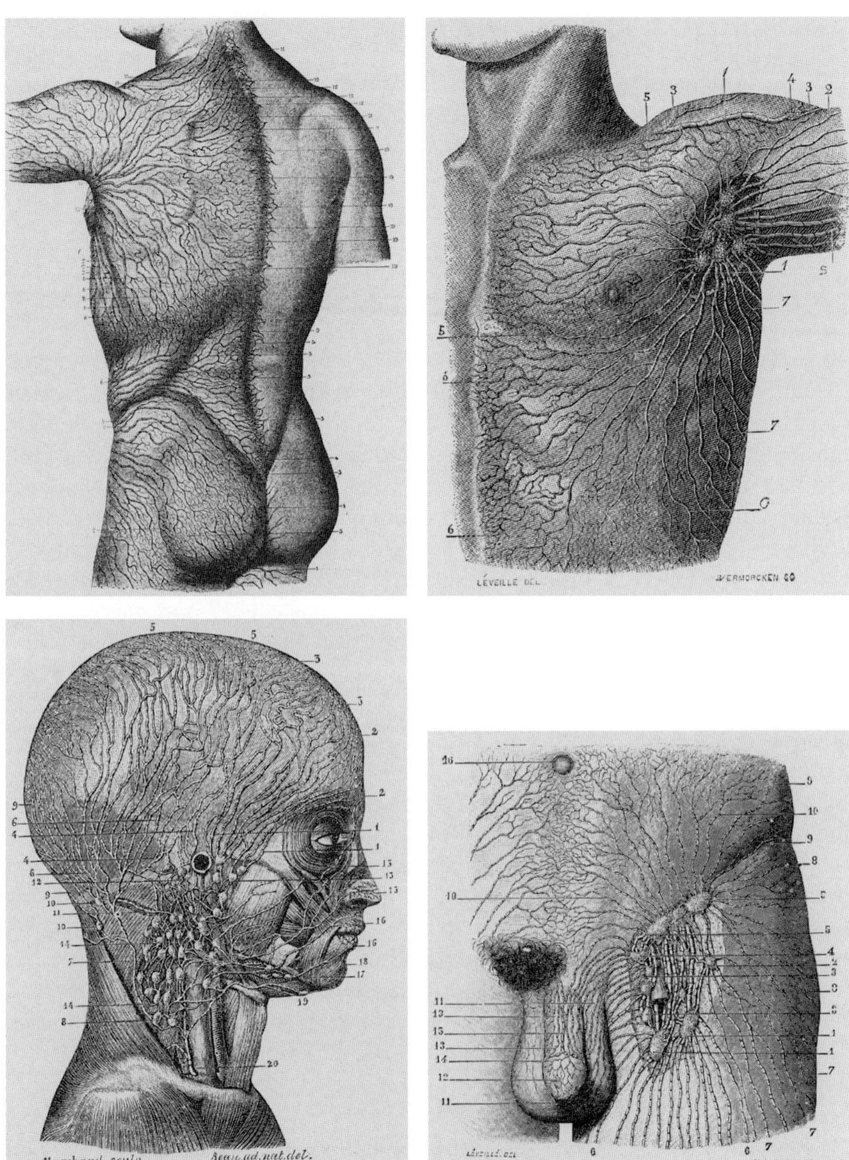

Figure 2.3 Sappey's drawings of lymphatic drainage

Sappey's atlas contained detailed drawings of the lymphatic drainage of the skin and breast. He stated that channels did not cross the midline nor did they cross a horizontal line around the waist from the umbilicus anteriorly to L2 level posteriorly. These elegant drawings were accepted as correct for 100 years.

2.6 MICROSCOPIC DISCOVERIES

Von Recklinghausen discovered the lymphatic endothelial cell in 1862 and demonstrated that it could be stained black with silver nitrate.[56] In 1894 Reaut, Regaud[57] and Ranvier[58] showed that every lymphatic commences as a closed ampulla within connective tissue. Nerves in the walls of the lymphatic vessels were described by Kytmanoff in 1901.[59]

2.7 MARKING THE LYMPHATIC PATHWAYS FOR STUDY

To study the path of the lymphatic vessels various techniques were developed to make them visible to the examiner. These involved either distending them or opacifying them with a visible substance. Injections of such substances were made directly into arteries or into the interstitial tissue. Water, gelatin, wax, oil, Chinese ink, Prussian blue dye, carmine in suspension, mercury and even bacteria were used in this way. For early histological studies Chinese ink, bacteria and coloured gelatin were favoured, though for macroscopic study mercury or coloured dyes such as Prussian blue were used. The use of mercury in the study of the lymphatics was first described by Meckel[32] and was used by Cruikshank[52] and Mascagni[54], but the method was refined later by Sappey, who used it extensively.

2.7.1 Sappey's Method

Sappey's method for injecting the cutaneous lymphatics of cadavers involved the use of a drawn out glass tube to inject the skin.[15] This was attached via a flexible tube to a column of mercury 30–40 cm high and sometimes up to 80 cm in height. If successful, the lymphatic capillaries would fill within 30–60 seconds. The tube was then withdrawn to avoid rupture. Sometimes the trunk of a lymphatic vessel was injected directly. Following injection the tissues were left to dry in the horizontal position. This caused them to become transparent, so that the mercury in the lymphatic capillaries could then be seen shining through.

2.7.2 Gerota's Method

Gerota modified Sappey's approach by injecting coloured materials such as absolute black, cinnabar and Prussian blue rather than mercury.[60] The advantage of this modification was that the study could be performed on the living as well as the dead. Prussian blue was the preferred dye, made up in a solution of turpentine and sulphuric ether immediately prior to injection. As with Sappey's method the injection was made using a glass tube drawn out over a flame to a fine point. It was then attached to a 10–20 cc syringe. Gerota's method had the additional advantage over Sappey's method that it better defined draining lymphatic territories. Mercury tended to reveal extended networks due to the high injection pressures which were involved, and paradoxically the finer lymphatic capillaries distended more with mercury than did the collecting vessels because the latter had more resilient walls with a muscle cell layer and more elastic fibres. Gerota's method, performed at low pressures, showed the vessels at closer to their true volume and was thus a more physiological mapping procedure (Figure 2.4).

2.8 THE TWENTIETH CENTURY

In the early 1900s Bartels used modifications of Gerota's method to make important contributions to the study of lymphatic drainage in man.[61] Later, with the discovery of X-rays, new methods became available to study lymphatic vessels in the living human. In the 1930s a colloidal preparation of thorium dioxide, Thorotrast, was developed. This was used *in vivo* and in postmortem studies. Gray in particular produced excellent postmortem demonstrations of

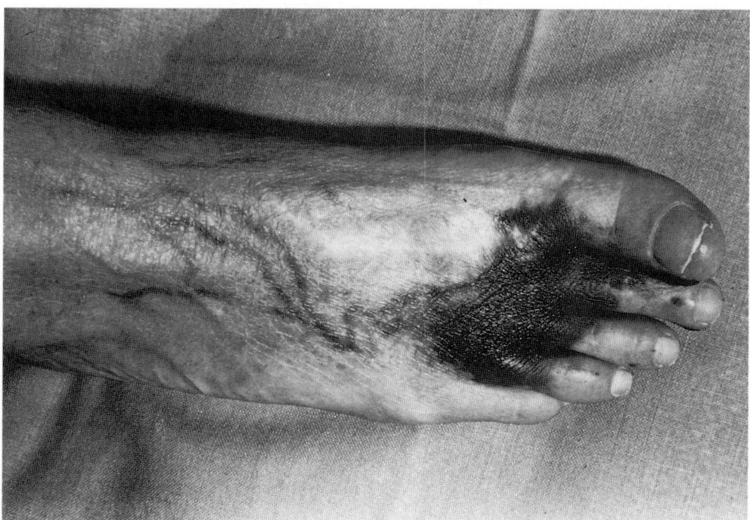

Figure 2.4 Blue dye in lymph vessels

Blue dye has been injected intradermally on the dorsum of the foot at the base of the toes. The dye enters the lymphatic capillaries and can be seen passing in several lymphatics along the dorsum of the foot towards the ankle. This was the basis of Gerota's method of studying the lymphatics.

the lymphatics using this method.[62] Unfortunately it was discovered that Thorotrast caused blood dyscrasias and malignant haemangioendothelioma of the liver and its use was discontinued.[63] At about the same time Hudack and McMaster first began using vital dyes *in vivo*.[64] The dye was injected into the tissues and thus entered the lymphatic capillaries, indirectly giving information on the lymphatic drainage of the tissues so injected. There was some application of this method to the study of clinical problems, and later many surgeons used this approach preoperatively as an aid to identifying draining lymph nodes for elective lymphadenectomy.[65, 66]

The technique of X-ray contrast lymphangiography was developed in 1952 by Kinmonth in England and became the standard method of examining the lymphatic system in man *in vivo*.[67] His technique involved injecting Patent Blue dye subcutaneously on the dorsum of the hand or foot to highlight a lymphatic trunk which he would then dissect down to and cannulate before injecting a radio-opaque dye. This injection was thus directly into the lymphatic trunk. It was used in many thousands of patients and good quality radiographs of the lymphatic collecting vessels and the draining lymph nodes were obtained. Much of the detailed knowledge we now have of human lymphatic drainage patterns came from such studies.[68] The method used large volumes of contrast material injected directly into lymphatic capillaries with the aim of opacifying as much of the system as possible. It was most often used to assess the possibility of metastatic involvement of lymph nodes, and to do this as many nodes as possible needed to be opacified. However, this high-volume, high-pressure injection method was not physiological and this limitation paved the way for the development of a tracer method.

2.9 LYMPHOSCINTIGRAPHY

In the early 1950s the tracer method, which became known as lymphoscintigraphy, was first used in humans.[69] It has since become the standard technique used for lymphatic mapping studies in man.

Chapter 3

LYMPHATIC MAPPING USING LYMPHOSCINTIGRAPHY

3.1 RADIOCOLLOIDS AND LYMPHATIC PHYSIOLOGY

3.1.1 The Effect of Particle Size

The fate of particles injected interstitially depends principally on their size (see Figure 3.1).

• 1–2 nanometres

Particles up to 1 or 2 nanometres in diameter will tend to enter the venous blood system directly.

• 5–25 nanometres

Particles of this size enter lymphatic capillaries via the gaps between cell junctions and the intercellular clefts formed by overlapping cells, which even when closed measure 10 to 25 nanometres across. The uptake rate of particles into lymphatic capillaries is independent of particle size within the range 6 to 18 nanometres, presumably because of these gaps and clefts.[40] Above this size the interstitial elastin matrix begins to pose a barrier to the movement of particles and their uptake into lymphatic capillaries.

• 25–100 nanometres

Particles up to 75 nanometres in diameter may gain entry into the lymphatic lumen by pinocytosis.[33,34] Such particles can enter the invaginations in the outer wall of the endothelial cell (see Figure 1.1) and then be transported in vesicles through the cell cytoplasm to the luminal wall before being emptied into the lumen of the lymphatic capillary. As mentioned earlier, this vesicular movement is not all in one direction, as particles can also enter the lymphatic

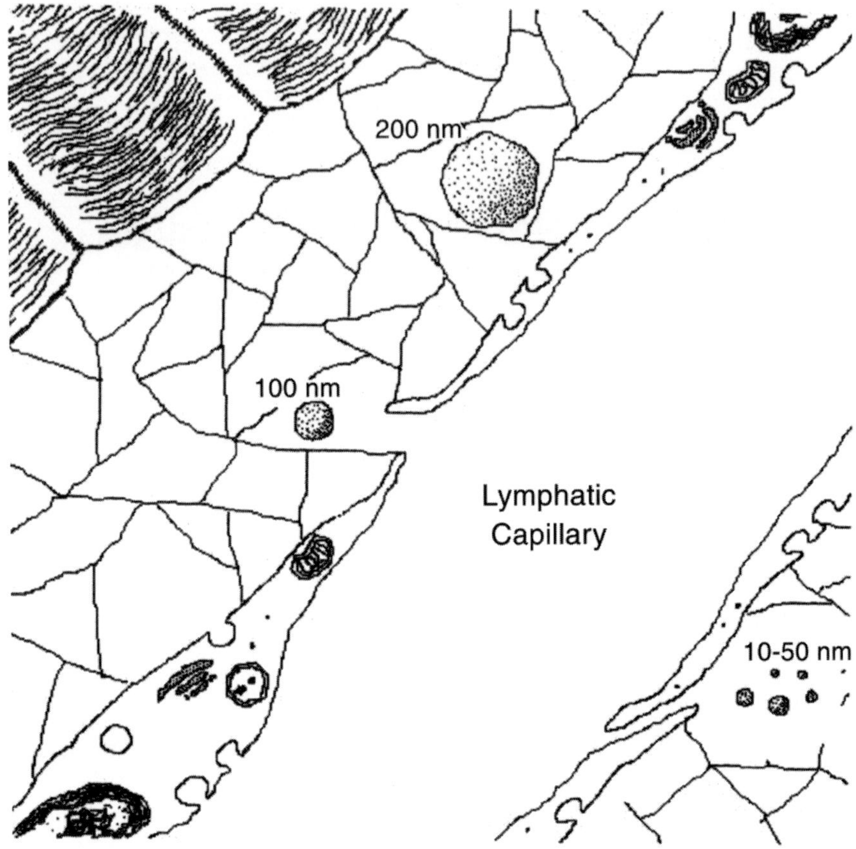

Figure 3.1 The fate of radiocolloids after intradermal injection

There is ready access to the lymphatic capillary lumen for particles in the 5–25 nanometre range via the clefts between the endothelial cells which constitute the wall of the lymphatic vessel. The separation between the cells at these junction points is 10 to 25 nanometres. Some large particles will gain entry, as larger gaps are intermittently opened up when the elastin fibrils attached to the outside of the endothelial cells are tensed by movement of the tissues. Some particles up to 75 nanometres in diameter will be transported across the endothelial cell to the lumen of the lymphatic capillary in the vesicles which are abundant in the walls of the endothelial cells. These form pinocytic vesicles which can then empty their contents into the capillary lumen. Particles between 50–100 nanometres however are beginning to have difficulty moving through the interstitial lattice of elastin and collagen fibrils and fibres. The larger particles over 100 nanometres tend to be trapped in the interstitium with only a few gaining entry into the lymphatic capillary via the occasional large gaps which occur in the endothelial wall. These can reach 2000–3000 nanometres in diameter in some circumstances but these large gaps are not common.

endothelial cell from the lumen of the capillary via these caveolae and accumulate in cytoplasmic vacuoles (see Figure 1.3). It is thus not clear what the net effect of pinocytosis is on the transport of particles from the interstitium through the lymphatic endothelial cell into the lumen of lymphatic capillaries.

The matrix of reticular and elastin fibres which makes up the connective tissue surrounding the lymphatic capillaries also begins to pose a physical barrier to particles in the 70 to 100 nanometre range. Above this diameter particles will find this connective tissue lattice increasingly difficult to penetrate (Figure 3.1). Some particles in the 25–100 nanometre range will gain entry into the lymphatic capillaries via the very large gaps which can occasionally be seen between cells de novo and via the effects of movement and tension in the soft tissues (see Figure 1.9). Such movement causes tension on the elastin fibrils which attach the outside of the endothelial cells to the collagen fibres of the connective tissue matrix, causing the gaps between the lymphatic endothelial cells to open.[42]

- 100–1000 nanometres

Larger particles (hundreds of nanometres) will remain trapped in the interstitial space for some time.[70–74] Such large particles rely on mechanical factors to open up the gaps in intercellular junctions, as mentioned above. Such mechanical factors can include an increase in interstitial fluid pressure, as well as movement and twisting of the soft tissues.

3.1.2 Flow Rates of Radiocolloids in Lymphatics

Many factors influence the rate of clearance of radiocolloids from their injection site. The larger the colloid, the slower its clearance after interstitial injection. The rate of flow of Tc99m-human serum albumin in lymphatics following intradermal injection has recently been measured.[75] This material is a non-particulate tracer. Nathanson found the average flow rate in a total of 17 patients was 10.4 ± 7.3 cm/min. We have measured the movement of 99mTc-antimony sulphide colloid through the lymphatic capillaries following intradermal injection in 198 patients with primary melanoma sites on various parts of the body. We found an average flow rate of 4.4 cm/min.[41]

3.1.3 Factors Affecting Flow Rates of Radiocolloids in Lymphatics

3.1.3.1 *Injection site*

The rate of movement of colloid particles as they travel in lymphatic vessels to the draining lymph node fields appears to vary depending on the site of intradermal injection of the tracer. We initially measured how far the colloid particles travelled over a period of 10 minutes following intradermal injection of 99mTc antimony sulphide colloid.[76] The average speed at which the colloid moved was 1.6 cm/min for the arm, 3.1 cm/min for the forearm, 2.6 cm/min for the posterior trunk, 2.3 cm/min for the anterior trunk and 5.8 cm/min for the lower limb. There were limitations in the methodology of this initial study because patients who had activity present in their sentinel nodes at the end of the 10 minute dynamic acquisition were excluded, as were patients with no movement of tracer over 10 minutes.

Subsequently we have studied the lymph flow rate directly in 198 patients with melanoma.[41] The results of this study are shown in Table 3.1.

There are thus significant differences in lymph flow rates from the skin of different parts of the body. The fastest movement of the tracer through the lymphatic channels occurs from the leg, with the forearm having the next fastest flow rate (Figure 3.2). It is interesting that these skin areas also have the longest lymphatic paths to follow before they reach the draining node fields. Flow rates from the trunk were similar front and back, at about 30–40% of the flow rate from the lower limb (Figure 3.3 and Figure 3.4). The slowest rates of flow occurred from the skin of the head and neck and arm or shoulder. An absence of flow on the early dynamic images was most common for the shoulder or arm, the head and neck and the thigh (Figure 3.5).

Table 3.1 Lymph flow rate in different skin regions

Region	*Average lymph flow rate (cm/min)*
Head and neck	1.5
Anterior trunk	2.8
Posterior trunk	3.9
Arm and shoulder	2.0
Forearm and hand	5.5
Thigh	4.2
Leg or foot	10.2

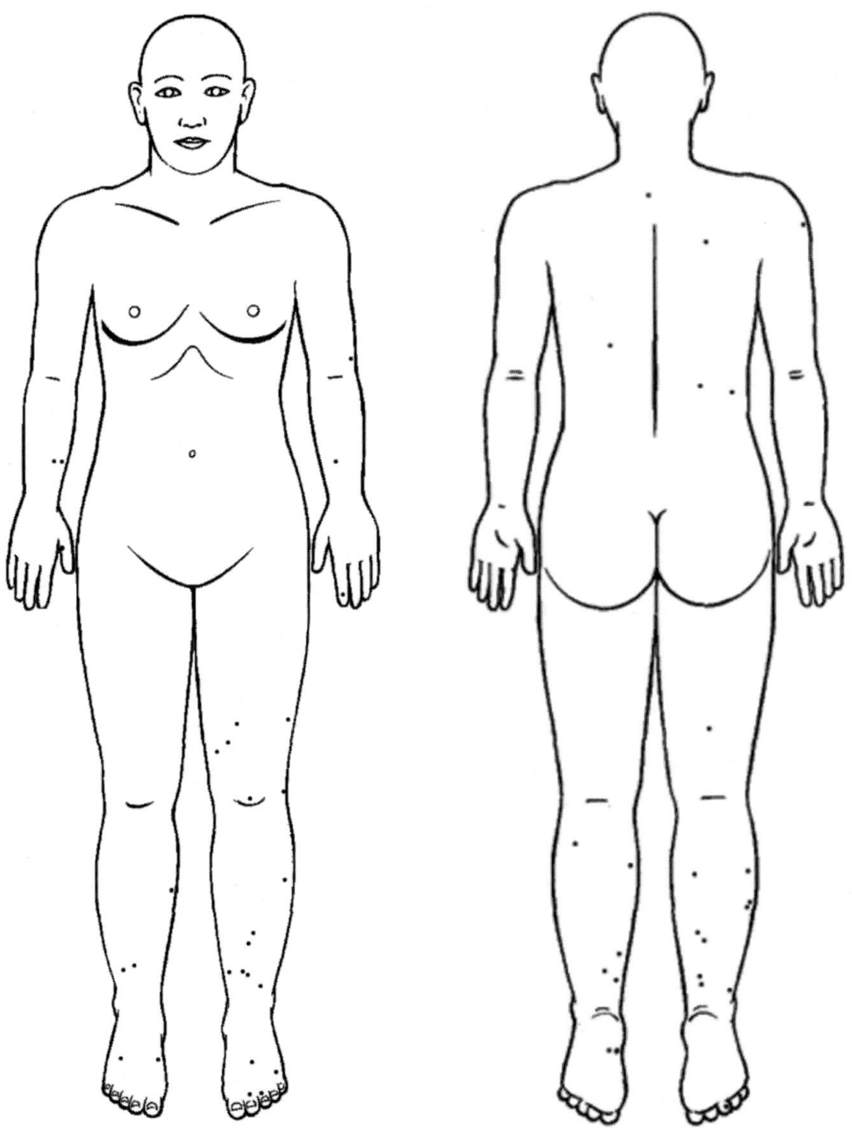

Figure 3.2 Sites which show high lymph flow rates >10 cm/min

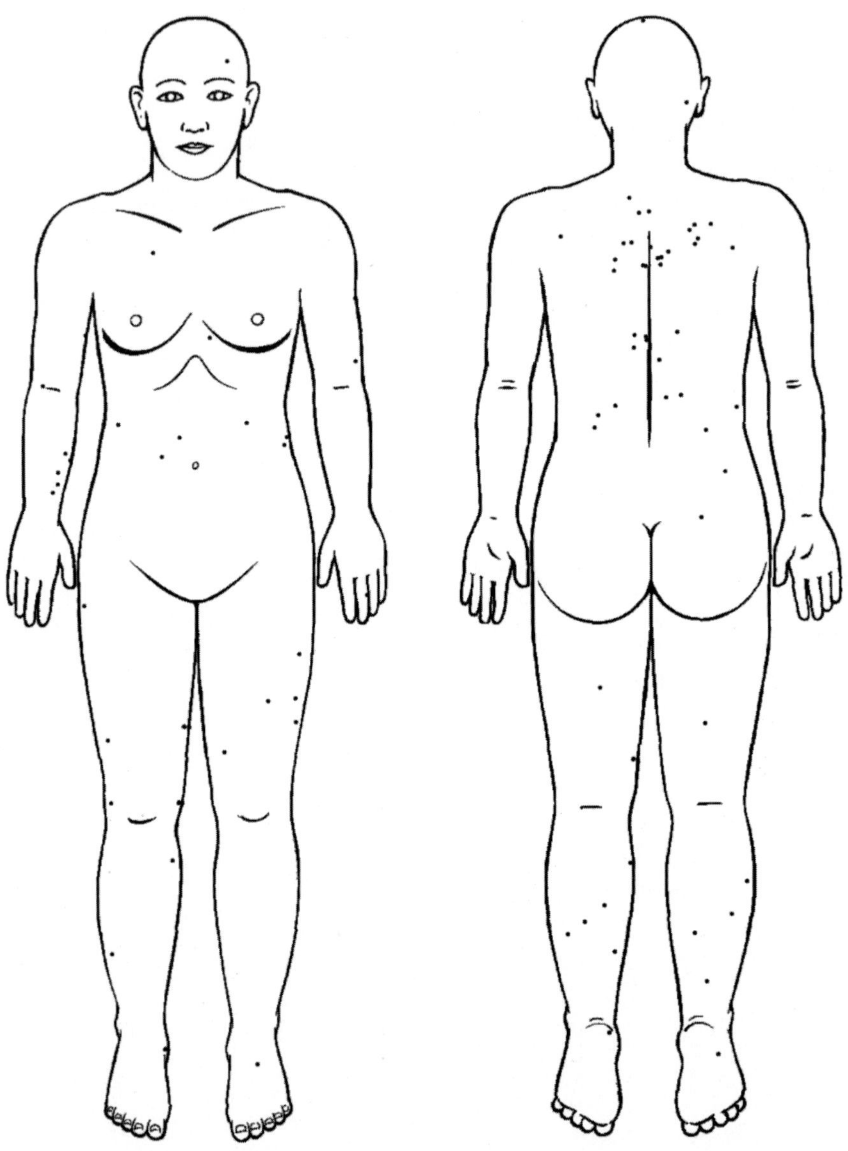

Figure 3.3 Skin sites from which there was lymphatic flow of 5–9 cm/min

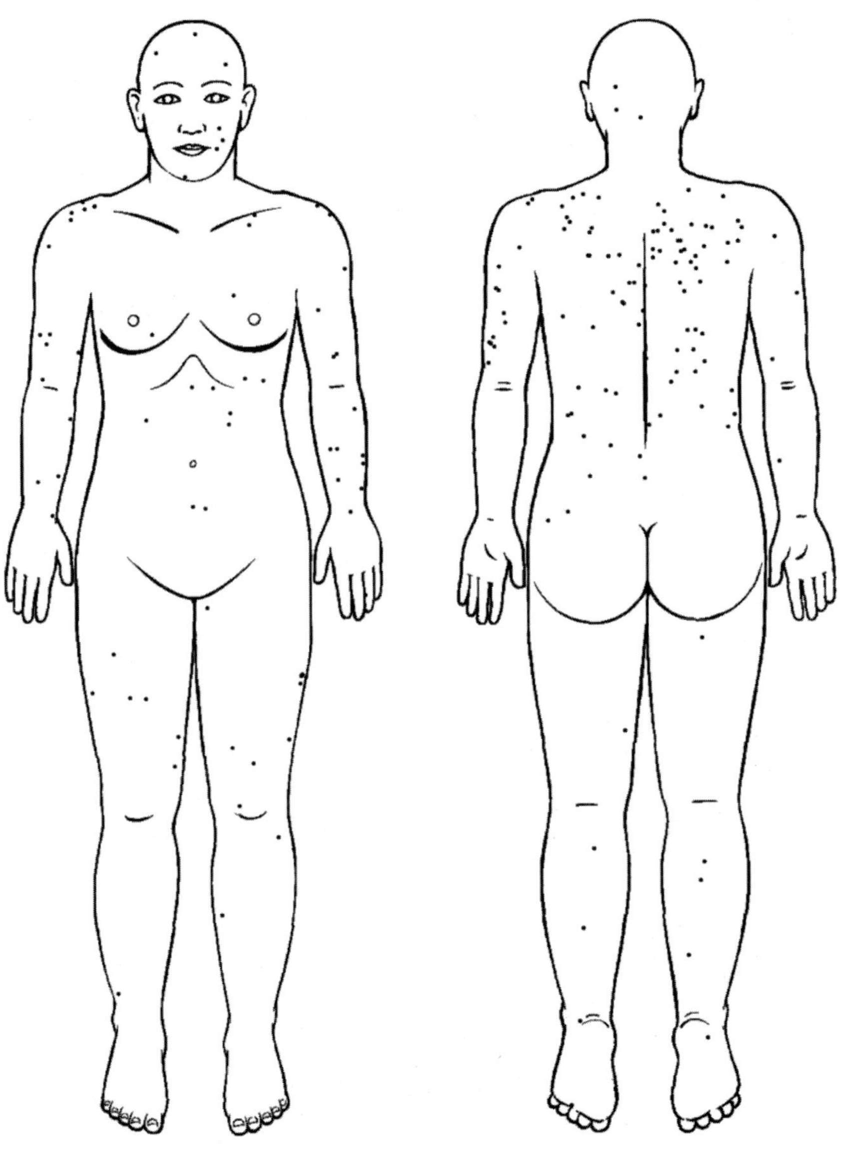

Figure 3.4 Skin sites from which there was lymphatic flow of 1–4 cm/min

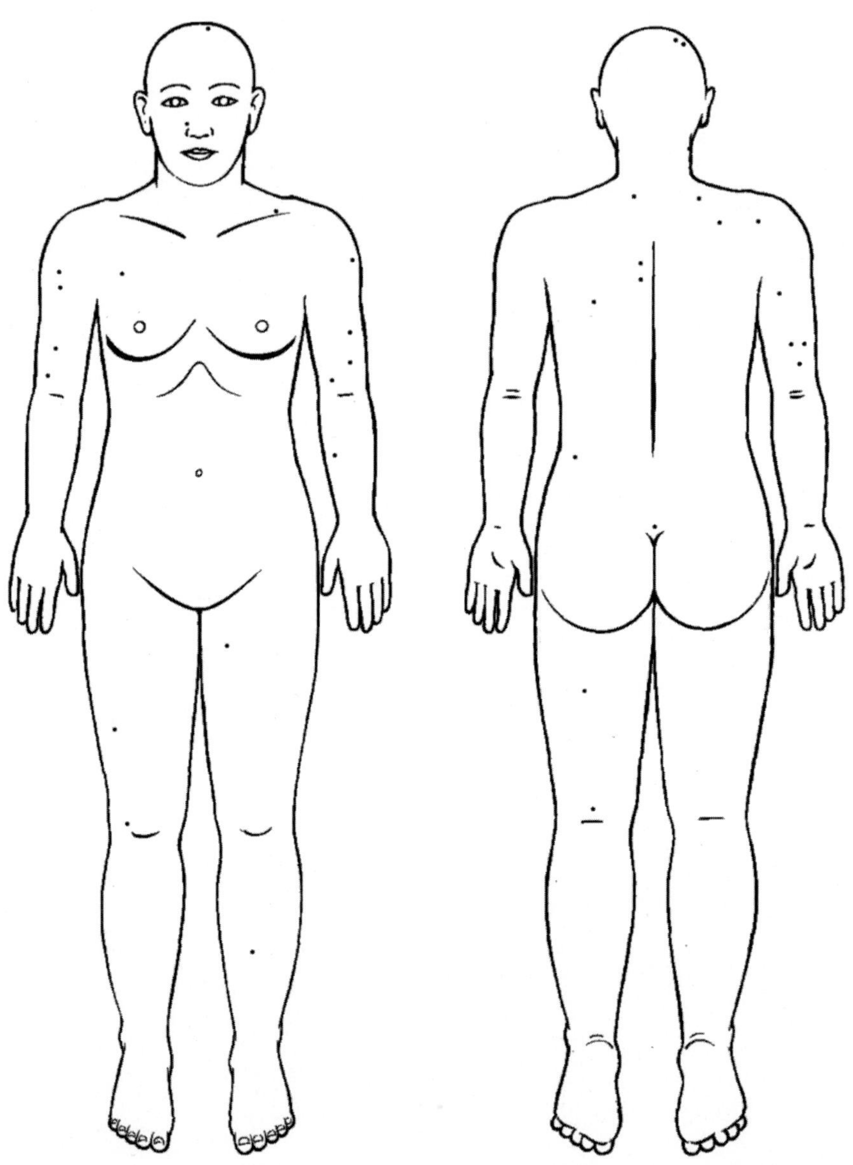

Figure 3.5 Skin sites from which there was no flow on dynamic imaging

3.1.3.2 *Interstitial pressure*

The volume of injected tracer will certainly affect uptake in lymphatic capillaries as a larger volume will increase interstitial pressure, thus greatly increasing tracer movement into the lymph vessels. An increase in interstitial pressure from 10 to 40 cm H_2O significantly increases the rate of uptake of particles into the terminal lymphatics, and also increases the production of lymph fluid and the volume of lymphatic flow.[40] When performing lymphoscintigraphy, the volume of injectate will therefore be an important factor in determining the rate of movement of tracer into the lymphatic capillaries. This fact can be used to partially overcome the disadvantages of using colloids with large particle sizes such as 99mTc-sulphur colloid. If larger volumes of tracer are used, more of the tracer will migrate through the lymphatics. Increased injection pressure, however, does not increase net velocity of lymph flow and the increased volume of lymph flow in this circumstance appears to be achieved by dilatation of the lymphatic channels and the opening up of other lymphatic capillaries.[40]

This raises a potential problem when using large injection volumes during lymphoscintigraphy to locate sentinel lymph nodes, since the fundamentals of the tracer method demand that the system under study not be perturbed by the study itself. This is why we favour small (0.05 ml) volumes of 99mTc antimony sulphide colloid at each injection site to allow the true lymphatic physiology to be studied and to minimise any disturbance of the system. In the breast, where the connective tissue matrix is less dense, the resistance to injection is much lower than in the skin. We have therefore increased the volume of injectate slightly for mammary lymphoscintigraphy from 0.1 ml to 0.2 ml to more closely approximate the interstitial pressures achieved in the skin. If large volumes are used, however, there is the potential for lymphatic channels away from the lesion, and thus the injection site, to open up and drain colloid to nodes which do not normally drain the primary tumour site.

Large injection volumes (1 ml per injection site) have been used in breast lymphoscinitigraphy with the aim of ensuring visualisation of the sentinel nodes in the axilla when using filtered 99mTc sulphur colloid.[77] This does reduce the problem of lack of migration of the colloid when small volume injections (0.05 to 0.1 ml) of this colloid are used, but it raises the concerns mentioned above. There has even been one recent report of using 4 intramammary injections of 4 ml each for a total volume of 16 ml![78] Such large volumes are non-physiological and may cause entry of colloid particles into lymph channels which under normal conditions would not drain the tumour site. Although such approaches may lead to 'hot' nodes being found in 90% of patients using microfiltered 99mTc sulphur colloid, serious doubts must be raised as to whether the 'hot' nodes found would actually drain the tumour site under physiological conditions and thus whether these are in fact true sentinel nodes. Inaccurate identification of nodes, which under physiological conditions would not receive lymph from the tumour site being studied, defeats the purpose of sentinel node biopsy.

3.1.3.3 *Inflammation*

Inflammation will also increase the production and rate of lymph flow. This is commonly present in the skin when lymphoscintigraphy is performed following excision-biopsy of the primary melanoma. Experience suggests that this does not cause any change in the ability of lymphoscintigraphy to detect the true sentinel node. In fact there may even be an advantage in performing lymphoscintigraphy in this situation, as the enhanced lymph flow may actually facilitate identification of the sentinel node. In breast cancer we normally perform lymphoscintigraphy before removal of the primary tumour and there is usually no inflammation present at the time of the study.

3.1.3.4 *Movement of the tissues*

Having the patient exercise the limb after injection of radiocolloid will increase the rate of flow of tracer through the lymphatic channels, as will massaging the injection site. However, imaging protocols in melanoma patients require immediate dynamic imaging which must be performed with the patient lying still under the gamma camera, thus this option is not practical in most patients undergoing cutaneous lymphoscintigraphy. However, it does not seem to be necessary in the skin as lymphatic channels are routinely visualised on dynamic imaging. Exercise and gentle massage are nevertheless a useful adjunct when injecting blue dye preoperatively, and both can be used with good effect in patients having a sentinel node biopsy procedure using a gamma detection probe without lymphoscintigraphy. Massage is a particularly useful manoeuvre in patients undergoing breast lymphoscintigraphy as the intramammary injections are usually given under ultrasound guidance and dynamic imaging is thus delayed for a few minutes. Over this period it is very important to have the patient gently massage the breast around the sites of injection to enhance movement of the tracer through the breast lymphatics.

3.1.3.5 *Previous surgery*

Previous lymphatic or lymph node surgery has a profound effect on lymphatic drainage. There may simply be a decrease in the number of lymph channels and lymph nodes seen, progressing through to overt lymphoedema with no channels, dermal backflow and no uptake whatsoever in lymph nodes (Figure 3.6). It has been appreciated for some time that lymphoscintigraphy following wide

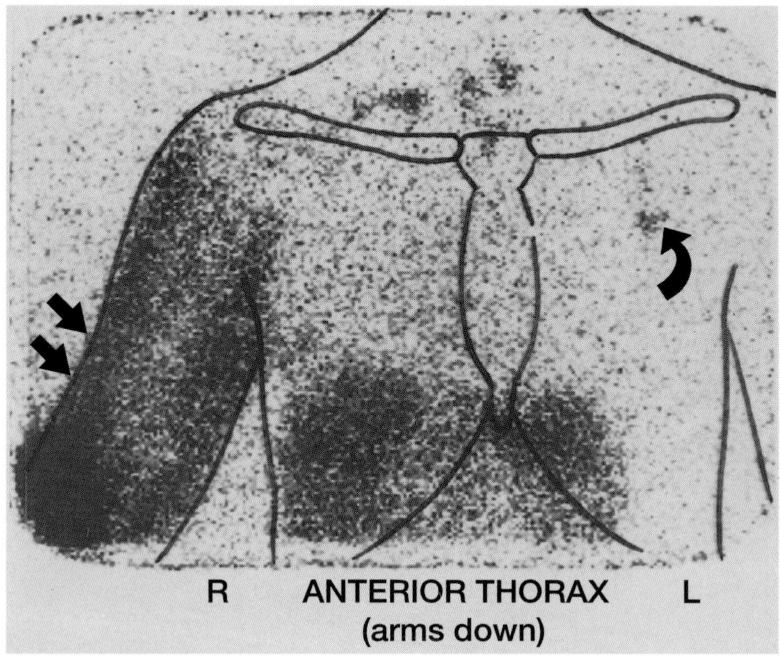

Figure 3.6 Surgery alters lymphatic flow patterns

This woman had an elective radical dissection of her right axilla for carcinoma of the right breast several years prior to presenting with a melanoma on the right arm. There were no dominant lymph channels on the dynamic phase of the study and on delayed imaging there was obvious dermal backflow (arrows) in the right arm and no nodes were seen in the right axilla. Tracer was seen passing across the neck to a node in the left axilla (curved arrow). Surgery causes a marked disruption of lymphatic flow patterns and this disruption is unpredictable. It is preferable to perform lymphatic mapping prior to any intervention whether it is surgery or radiotherapy.

local excision in patients with melanoma is unreliable, often resulting in no migration of the radiocolloid in the disrupted lymphatics. Early reports are also appearing suggesting that performing lymphoscintigraphy in patients with breast cancer after they have undergone lumpectomy or radiation therapy causes false negative sentinel node biopsies with 'skip' metastases being found in non-sentinel nodes.[79] Therefore in patients with melanoma we perform lymphoscintigraphy prior to wide local excision of the biopsy site and in breast cancer patients before lumpectomy. There are two good reasons for this approach: (1) wide local excision and breast cancer lumpectomy will have an unpredictable effect on the patterns of lymphatic drainage, and (2) surgery the day after lymphoscintigraphy removes the skin and breast tissue which has received the highest dose of radiation from the radiocolloid. This can be as high as 0.45 Gy if there is no migration of the tracer.

3.1.3.6 *Metastatic involvement*

If lymphatic channels are partially or completely blocked by metastatic tumour deposits this will certainly decrease or even totally block the flow of radiocolloid through the system and may decrease the number of nodes visualised on delayed scans (Figure 3.7). This is usually not a practical problem when performing cutaneous lymphatic mapping to locate sentinel nodes, as this is only performed in patients who do not have clinically palpable metastatic lymph nodes. It is a potentially more relevant problem with breast lymphoscintigraphy however, because clinical detection of metastatic disease in axillary nodes is notoriously difficult.

3.1.4 Uptake and Retention in Lymph Nodes

Foreign particles carried with the lymph flow are mostly phagocytosed in the lymph nodes.[80] Colloid particles are phagocytosed after they have been recognised as foreign or have been coated with opsonins and thus recognised. The phagocytic cells are macrophages, which are concentrated especially in the subcapsular and medullary sinuses.[23] The surface charge of the particle and the agent used as a stabiliser in the production of the colloid will affect the rate of phagocytosis.[81] The rate of opsonisation can also be markedly increased by the use of sterically stabilised nanocolloids.[82] The rate of phagocytosis of such colloids is greatly increased, so that up to 40% of the injected dose is trapped in the draining lymph nodes. Uptake in the draining lymph nodes can also be increased by using receptor-binding radiotracers.[83]

Of the tracers which have been used clinically for lymphoscintigraphy the highest levels of uptake in the draining lymph nodes have been achieved with colloidal gold and 99mTc antimony sulphide colloid. Two hours following interstitial injection, uptake in lymph nodes averages 8% and 6% of the injected dose respectively for these two agents.[73] For other small particle size colloids such as stannous colloid and rhenium sulphide colloid uptake is 1–2%. Colloids with larger particles such as sulphur colloid and albumin colloid only show approximately one-third of this uptake in the lymph nodes.[80] Using 99mTc-nanocolloid, Kapteijn found an average of 0.69% of the injected dose in sentinel lymph nodes and 0.23% in non-sentinel second tier nodes 24 hours following intradermal injection.[84]

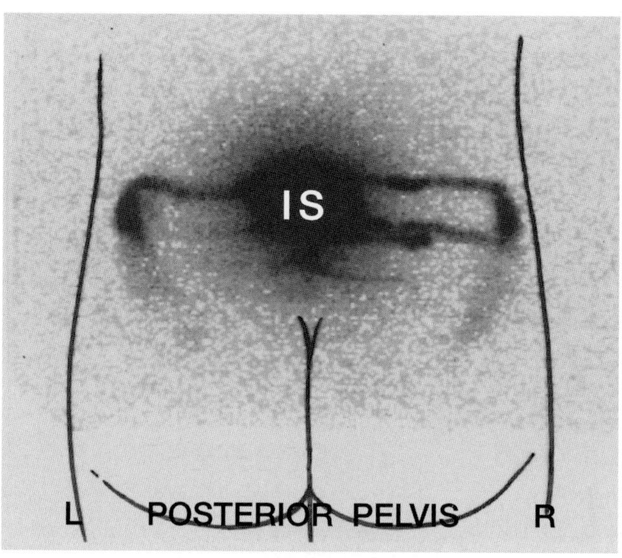

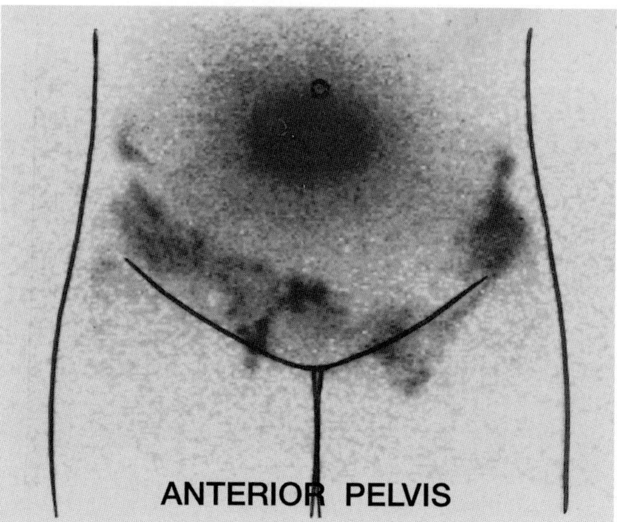

Figure 3.7 Metastases in channels and nodes will affect lymphoscintigraphy

This patient had obvious clinically involved nodes in both groins and in-transit metastases were seen in the skin along the line of the lymph channels. However, on the dynamic images, channels are seen passing from the injection site (IS) on the mid low back around to the groin bilaterally. Flow through the channels was slow in this patient and the nodes were poorly visualised on both the early and late scans.

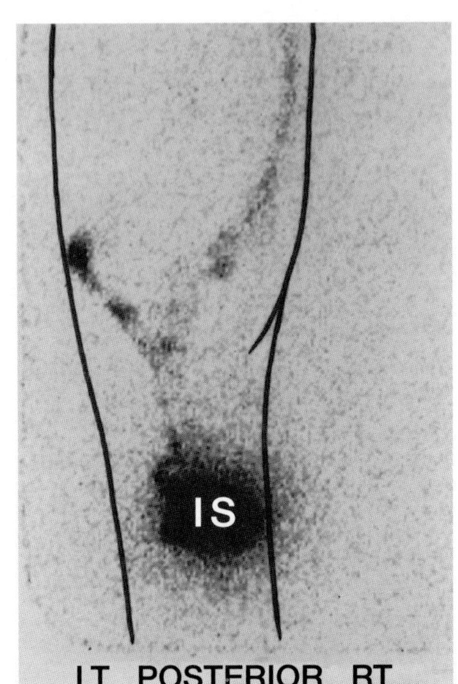

A

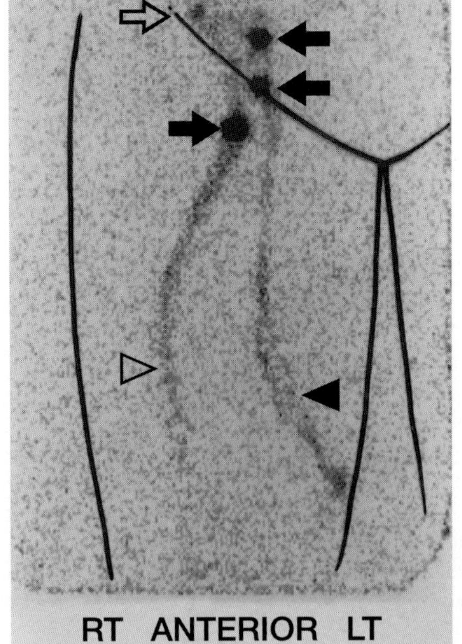

B

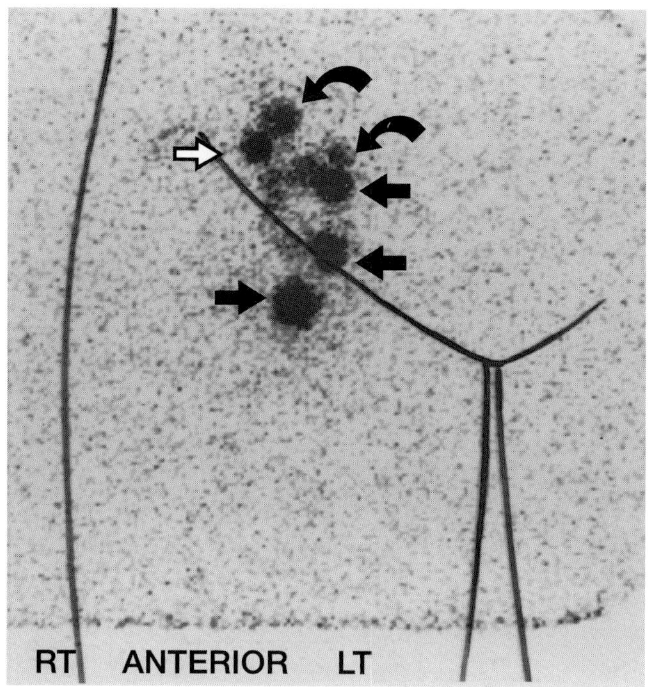

C

Figure 3.8 Multiple sentinel nodes and second tier nodes in the groin

A: Two dominant channels are seen passing from the injection site (IS) on the back of the right leg above the ankle up the medial and lateral sides of the leg towards the right groin. B: The early dynamic phase over the groin shows these channels reach three sentinel nodes in the groin (arrows). There are two channels medially (arrowhead) which pass up together to meet two nodes, and what appears to be a single channel laterally (open arrowhead) that reaches a sentinel node and appears to then pass rapidly onwards to a higher node laterally in the groin (open arrow). In this situation when a node appears early on dynamic imaging, even though it may look as though it is receiving tracer which has passed through a sentinel node, it should be marked as a possible sentinel node so that the situation can be checked at the time of surgery. In this patient there were in fact 4 sentinel nodes, as a separate lymph channel was found bypassing the inferolateral sentinel node to directly enter the node higher in the groin laterally (open arrow). C: On delayed imaging this node had similar activity to several adjacent second tier nodes (curved arrows) and it would not be possible to distinguish this node from the second tier nodes with a gamma probe or with any count threshold technique. High quality lymphoscintigraphy is needed to ensure that these patients have an accurate and complete sentinel node biopsy procedure.

The retention of 99mTc antimony sulphide colloid in the sentinel node is excellent and even at 24 hours post-injection the sentinel nodes invariably remain by far the most radioactive nodes.[85] This is especially true in the axilla, though even in the groin following lower limb injections, where activity in second tier nodes is more common, the sentinel node usually remains the hottest node (Figure 3.8).

We recently examined the frequency with which 99mTc antimony sulphide colloid was seen in second tier lymph nodes, i.e. those beyond the sentinel node, during routine lymphoscintigraphy.[86] We found marked regional variations in this frequency. Second tier nodes were apparent in all patients with melanoma sites on the leg and thigh, and in the axilla with hand and forearm melanomas, but were much less commonly seen in the axilla with trunk or arm melanomas. Drainage to second tier lymph nodes also occurred less often in patients with melanoma sites on the head and neck. The incidence of second tier drainage was compared to the speed of lymph flow and there was a very high correlation found, indicating that this is a major factor associated with this phenomenon.

If the lymph nodes are replaced by metastatic tissue (Figure 3.9) then it is theoretically possible that radiocolloid will not accumulate in the node and that a sentinel node could be missed (Figure 3.7). In practice this does not appear to be a significant problem since the sentinel node biopsy procedure is usually not performed when there are palpable nodal metastases. It remains possible, however, that non-palpable sentinel nodes containing metastasis could be missed in this way.

3.2 RADIOPHARMACEUTICALS FOR LYMPHOSCINTIGRAPHY

3.2.1 The First Radiocolloid for Lymphoscintigraphy

The concept of lymphoscintigraphy was developed by Walker, and reported in 1950.[87] The original radiocolloid used for lymphoscintigraphy was gold-198 colloid which had a very desirable uniform colloid size of 5 to 10 nanometres, however the beta emissions associated with this tracer caused very high and therefore undesirable radiation doses at the site of injection.[69]

3.2.2 The 99m-Technetium Labelled Radiocolloids

The development of 99mTc with its high photon flux and low radiation dose spurred the development of radiocolloids labelled with this isotope. 99mTc-sulphur colloid with a range of particle size of 50 to 2000 nanometres and with an average size of 300 nanometres was used first, but the large particle size and slow clearance from the injection site encouraged the development of techne-

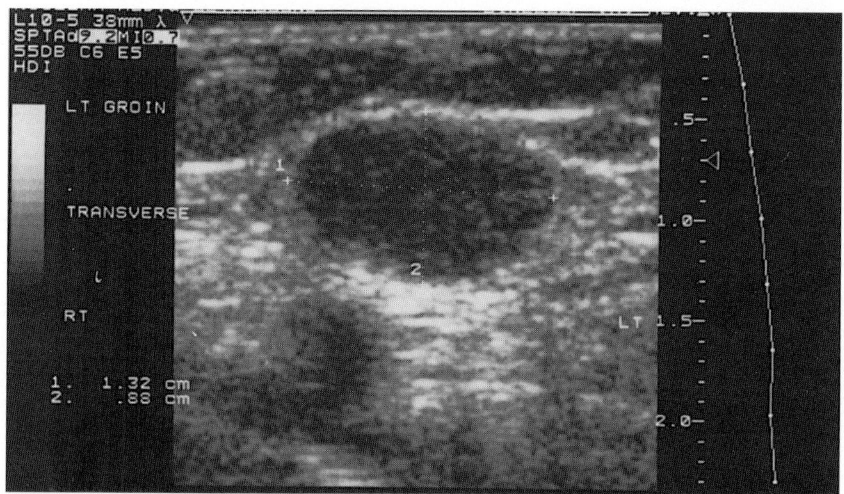

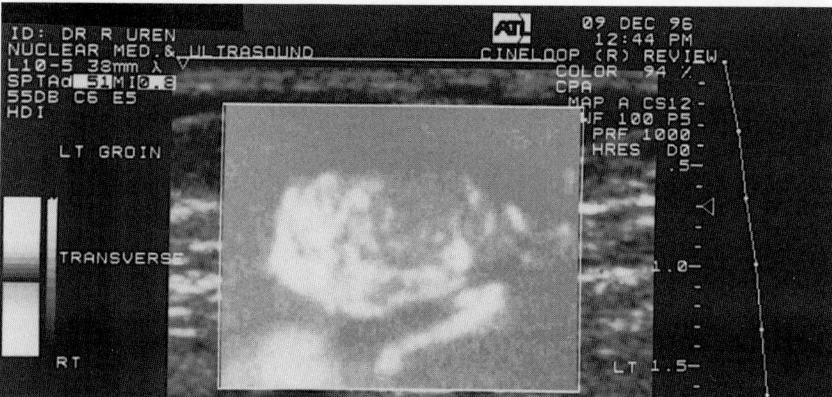

Figure 3.9 Metastatic lymph nodes on ultrasound

A transverse ultrasound scan through a metastatic lymph node in the left groin using a high resolution 5–10 MHz probe (ATL Ultramark 9 HDI). Lymph nodes which are full of melanoma metastases are rounded in appearance with low level internal echoes on ultrasound examination. They also lose the normal hilar echoes and often have an increased vascular signature on colour doppler imaging or colour power angiography. Nodes such as this would not be expected to accumulate radiocolloid in the normal way.

tium colloids with a smaller particle size. 99mTc-stannous phytate and 99mTc-antimony sulphide colloid were both investigated as agents for lymphoscintigraphy in humans.[71] In this study Kaplan concluded that 99mTc-antimony sulphide colloid was the agent of choice for lymphoscintigraphy and our experience supports this view. It migrates rapidly through the lymphatic vessels to the draining node field and yet there is excellent retention in the sentinel node for up to 24 hours. This allows the gamma probe to be effectively used at the time of surgery the day after lymphoscintigraphy.[85] It provides the most comprehensive map of the lymphatic system of the skin and is therefore the best agent to use, if available, as it accurately reflects the physiological lymphatic drainage in an individual patient.

Antimony sulphide colloid has particles of relatively uniform size, most with diameters in the 10–15 nanometres range although some do range up to 40 nanometres. This colloid is also very stable, with the particles remaining at their initial size for at least 5 hours. Such antimony sulphide colloid particles are an ideal size to pass freely into the lymphatic capillaries via the 10 to 25 nanometre clefts between overlapping cells (see Figures 1.8 and 3.1) and the intercellular gaps, which can be considerably larger than this. Good results can also be obtained using ultra-filtered 99mTc rhenium sulphur colloid which produces a significant number of particles in the 50 nanometre range.[80] Similarly 99mTc-nanocolloid which is a colloid of albumin, migrates well following intradermal injection and good scans are produced in most patients. This tracer has a range of particle size (3 to 80 nanometres) but 77% are less than 30 nanometres.[84] Other tracers which have been used include 99mTc human serum albumin colloid, 99mTc microaggregated albumin, 99mTc macroaggregated albumin and mouse antibodies labelled with 99mTc, though none of these appear to be as satisfactory as 99mTc-antimony sulphide colloid.

Tc-sulphur colloid has been widely used for many years, especially in the United States of America, and has a wide range of particle sizes as mentioned above with a mean of 300 nanometres. If the particles are pushed through a 0.2 micron filter, particles over 200 nanometres can effectively be removed, however the colloid must be used soon after filtering as the particle size increases slowly over a 5-hour period unlike antimony sulphide which has a stable particle size over this period. Such filtered sulphur colloid is favoured by some, as due to its larger size it tends to be retained well by the sentinel node.[88] This is in contrast to 99mTc-human serum albumin which as a non-particulate tracer migrates more rapidly on to second tier nodes and the systemic circulation. The size of the 99mTc-sulphur colloid particles remains a concern however, and does limit movement of this tracer into the lymphatic capillaries. Some of the smaller particles will freely enter the lymphatics via the intercellular clefts and gaps, but the larger range of particle sizes will have to rely on pinocytosis or physical factors to open up the gaps between endothelial cells before they can gain entry into the lymphatic lumen. As can be seen in Figure 3.1, particles in the 100–200 nanometres range find the elastin fibrous matrix of the interstitium poses a barrier to their free movement before they can even reach the lymphatic capillary. This means that there is greater retention of this tracer at the injection site and less migration to draining lymph nodes.

There is some evidence, at least *in vitro*, that the size of the particles in 99mTc-sulphur colloid is affected by the serum it comes in contact with in the patient.[81, 89] The particles may increase or decrease in size. This has not been shown with 99mTc antimony sulphide colloid or 99mTc albumin microcolloid.[80] The size distribution of 99mTc sulphur colloid is also significantly altered by the method of preparation.[90] The number of labelled particles in the less than 400 nanometre range is maximised by using a reduced heating time protocol (heat for 3 minutes and cool for 2 minutes, rather than the usual heat for 10 minutes and cool for 5 minutes). This results in just over 70% of the particles being less than 400 nanometres in diameter compared to about 40% with the longer protocol. It is also advantageous to use technetium from a generator with a long ingrowth time (i.e. greater than 72 hours), as this also favourably increases the particle size distribution profile towards the smaller particles. Filtered 99mTc sulphur colloid and 99mTc albumin colloid which have been passed through a 0.2 micron filter, however, do appear in clinical practice to be adequate for lymphoscintigraphy with reasonably rapid passage through the lymph channels and good retention in sentinel lymph nodes.[90] A recent study by Wong and colleagues suggested that particle size is not important in identifying the sentinel node and went so far as stating a preference for 99mTc sulphur colloid because there was less movement of this colloid onwards to second tier lymph nodes when compared to the other tracer they studied — 99mTc human serum albumin.[91] However, whenever 99mTc sulphur colloid has been directly compared to the smaller colloids such as antimony sulphide or nanocolloid of albumin it has been found that with sulphur colloid fewer channels are seen on dynamic images, fewer draining nodes fields per patient are seen and fewer sentinel nodes per node field are seen.[92] We remain concerned therefore that although a 'successful' sentinel node biopsy procedure may appear to be achieved using micro-filtered 99mTc sulphur colloid, not all true sentinel node will be detected in all patients.

99mTc-human serum albumin is frequently used in the USA for lymphoscintigraphy. Its non-particulate nature means that it enters the lymphatic capillaries rapidly via the intercellular clefts and gaps and does show rapid movement through the lymphatic channels.[75] However, because of its non-particulate nature, it may move rapidly on from the sentinel node to second tier nodes, which is a significant disadvantage when the purpose of lymphoscintigraphy is to locate the sentinel lymph nodes.[88] Sometimes it passes completely through the sentinel node so that on delayed lymphoscintigraphic scans no activity is seen in the sentinel nodes at all.[90]

The number of particles may influence the rate of movement from the injection site. Too many particles could saturate transport and lymphatic uptake mechanisms. For antimony sulphide colloid the number of particles in the usual preparation is in the order of 5×10^{13}/ml of solution With sulphur colloid there are about 10^{10} particles/ml with an average size of 300 nanometres. This variable is likely to have a greater effect on the transport of tracers which rely on cell mechanisms for their movement across the endothelial cell to the lymphatic lumen, for example the larger sized colloid particles which enter by pinocytosis. The number of particles is not likely to influence the entry of small particles such as antimony sulphide colloid or nanocolloid which pass mainly through the gaps and intercellular clefts without actually passing through the endothelial cell itself.

3.2.3 The Ideal Radiocolloid for Lymphatic Mapping

Based on the anatomical and physiological features of lymphatic capillaries and lymph nodes it is clear that the optimal particle size for interstitial lymphoscintigraphy with inert colloids is a diameter of 10 to 25 nanometres, so that the tracer can freely enter the lymphatic system but also be well retained in the draining lymph nodes (see Figure 1.8 and 3.1). Antimony sulphide colloid has most of its particles in this range, is also very stable in particle size over a 5-hour period and does not change its particle size on contact with the patient's serum. It also has excellent retention in the draining sentinel nodes. This is thus the best tracer (at present) to use for lymphatic mapping, if it is available. Nanocolloid labelled with 99mTc also gives good results since it has a large percentage of its particles in the desired size range.[84] In clinical practice, colloids of 99mTc sulphur colloid and 99mTc albumin colloid which have been passed through a 0.2 micron filter also appear adequate for high quality cutaneous lymphoscintigraphy.[93] We would counsel, however, that if antimony sulphide colloid or nanocolloid are available these should be used in preference to sulphur colloid and albumin colloid, as there remains significant doubt that all true sentinel nodes will be identified when using the latter two agents.

3.2.4 New 99mTc-labelled Tracers for Lymphatic Mapping

In an effort to further improve visualisation of lymphatic channels and sentinel lymph nodes some novel approaches have recently been described. New radiotracers using receptor-binding agents[83] or surface engineered nanospheres to increase phagocytosis in the regional lymph nodes[82] have been developed. Vera et al. have developed a non-particulate receptor-binding radiotracer which has excellent retention in the sentinel nodes, thus potentially offering the advantages of both rapid flow through lymph channels of the non-particulate agents such as human serum albumin and the good node retention of the particulate agents such as antimony sulphide colloid.[83] Moghimi et al. have used co-polymers to sterically stabilise nanospheres.[82] This dramatically increases the opsonisation of these agents in the lymph nodes so that up to 40% of the injected dose is trapped in sentinel node macrophages. Such a high percentage of the injected dose reaching draining lymph nodes also suggests that clearance from the injection site has been enhanced, perhaps by an increase in lymphatic capillary uptake of these agents through their opsonisation and active transport into the capillary by pinocytosis. Developments such as these may lead to better tracers for lymphoscintigraphy in the future.

3.3 RADIATION DOSIMETRY

When 99mTc radiopharmaceuticals are injected into the interstitial space the radiation dosimetry depends upon the rate of clearance of the tracer from the point of injection. Clearance of radiocolloids from the interstitial space is quite slow and thus there is a significant radiation dose delivered to the site of injection. A lesser dose is received by the lymph nodes, which drain the point of injection, and a very small dose is received by the reticuloendothelial system (RES), particularly the liver which ultimately traps the colloid particles after they reach the blood stream.

Bronskill measured the width of the injection site and the normalised count rate following intramuscular injection of 99mTc antimony sulphide colloid in the subcostal area.[94] This allowed an estimate of the clearance of tracer from the injection site over time. He found a biological half clearance time from this injection site of 20.6 hours. This meant that 5 hours after injection, 84.5% of the activity remained at the injection site, 2% was in the draining internal mammary lymph nodes and the other 13.5% was in the RES, mainly the liver. From these data Bronskill calculated an absorbed dose at the centre of the injection site of 0.456 Gy for an injected activity of 20 MBq (45.6 rads for 0.5 mCi). He also estimated the absorbed dose for a typical lymph node to be less than 0.2 Gy. Biological half clearance times from other sites were also measured. These were found to be 5.2 hours for the web space between the first and second toes, 9.4 hours for the web space between the second and third fingers and greater than 36 hours for perianal injections. Maximum dose estimates for these areas were 75 mGy/MBq for the toe web space, 84 mGy/MBq for the finger web space and 43 mGy/MBq for the perianal area. Bronskill did not specifically measure the absorbed dose for the intradermal injection of this tracer.

Glass et al. did measure the washout half-times after intradermal injection for 99mTc albumin colloid, 99mTc human serum albumin and 99mTc sulphur colloid (both of the colloids had been filtered through a 0.2 micron filter).[93] They found half-times from the injection site averaged 7.5 ± 6.4 hours, 4.3 ± 1.4 hours and

13.9 ± 12.7 hours respectively for the three agents. These clearance half-times imply lower doses at the injection site than those calculated by Bronskill. If one assumes a worst case scenario of no migration of tracer from the injection site after intradermal injection, maximum absorbed doses using 5 MBq of 99mTc antimony sulphide colloid at each injection site would be in the order of 0.45Gy assuming a volume of distribution of 1 cc. This is below the threshold dose for deterministic radiation effects and thus no erythema or other effect should be observed. When lymphoscintigraphy is performed to locate the sentinel nodes preoperatively, with our protocol the injections are given intradermally around the melanoma excision-biopsy site or into the breast around the cancer the day before wide local excision of the biopsy site or lumpectomy of the breast cancer. The radiation dose at the injection site, which accounts for the majority of the absorbed dose, thus becomes irrelevant as this tissue is excised within 24 hours of tracer injection.

Chapter 4

LYMPHATIC MAPPING OF THE SKIN

4.1 THE FIRST STUDIES

Using mercury injections in cadavers, Cruikshank[52] and Mascagni[54], and about 100 years later, Sappey[15] and his followers Poirier, Cuneo and Delamere[32], extensively documented the lymphatic drainage of the skin and other parts of the body. In the lower limb they detailed the superficial and deep lymphatic systems and described the common pathways which the lymphatic channels pursued to reach popliteal and inguinal nodes. They found that most of the lymphatic channels passed up the medial side of the lower limb and that the lateral channels also tended to pass towards the medial side of the limb.

In the upper limb, however, they suggested that the channels tended to follow one of three paths: an external group passing along the radial border of the forearm, an internal group following the ulnar border, and a middle group which ran parallel to the others but between them. They stated that some of the internal group reached the epitrochlear nodes and found some of the lateral group passing up over the shoulder to supraclavicular nodes and via the interpectoral groove to interpectoral nodes.

In reference to lymphatic drainage of the trunk Sappey stated 'In no part of the trunk or head have I seen any vessel spring from the side opposite to that to which it belonged'.[15] This was a concept embraced by most until the last few years. However, 100 years before Sappey's work was published Mascagni stated that 'lymphatic vessels of the right side of the lumbar and dorsal regions may arise from the left side and vice versa'.[54] Sappey simply declared that Mascagni was in error. We now know Mascagni was correct. Poirier, Cuneo and Delamere also realised that there were ambiguities in truncal drainage pathways in some situations.[32] They described anterior, posterior and lateral lymphatic territories on the thorax but conceded that this division was artificial, as the limits of these territories were indistinct. They also documented cases where draining vessels on the anterior thorax followed long curving paths above and below the breast to reach the axilla, though they believed all the anterior vessels terminated in 'the thoracic group' of axillary nodes. They did however describe 'accessory channels'.[32] These included: (1) a channel which passed from the upper anterior thorax superiorly over the clavicle to a supraclavicular node, (2) channels which originated a little distance from the midline but crossed it to reach the opposite axilla, and (3) a channel close to the midline which perforated the anterior intercostal space to pass into the internal mammary chain. We now recognise these as examples of the wide variation in lymphatic drainage of the trunk which can be seen in different patients.

Over the posterior thorax they recognised that drainage from the upper back was complex, with channels passing from the base of the neck to supraclavicular nodes, though again they were in error in believing that all other channels converged on the 'scapular group' of axillary nodes. The lateral group of channels was thought to pass superiorly to the 'thoracic group' of axillary nodes. Drainage from the gluteal regions was described as being around to the front and to the predictable groin nodes.

In the head and neck Poirier, Cuneo and Delamere, like Sappey, described a complex but predictable pattern of lymphatic drainage to node groups depending on the part of the skin injected. They also did not believe that drainage could occur across the midline or deviate significantly from these described pathways.

4.2 AMBIGUOUS DRAINAGE IGNORED

It is interesting to reflect that the ambiguities in lymphatic drainage of the skin, particularly from the trunk, were not pursued at the time. The work of those careful researchers who showed variations in the lymphatic drainage of the trunk was essentially ignored. Presumably the elegant illustrations in Sappey's atlas as well as his statements which denied the occurence of such ambiguous drainage persuaded most practitioners to accept his view. Most exclusively followed the strict teachings of Sappey until very recently. It has only been through increasing experience with lymphoscintigraphy that it has been confirmed that there are many variations in the lymphatic drainage of the skin in humans, with clinically predictable drainage from very few sites on the body.

4.3 THE TECHNIQUE OF CUTANEOUS LYMPHOSCINTIGRAPHY

4.3.1 Injecting the Tracer

For cutaneous lymphoscintigraphy the chosen radiopharmaceutical is administered by intradermal injection. The study should be performed in an air-conditioned environment with the temperature maintained at not less than 21–22°C. If the room is cold, lymph flow will be decreased and an unsuccessful study more likely. The procedure should be fully explained to the patient prior to commencing the study so that he or she is relaxed and comfortable about what is to happen. It is particularly important to warn the patient that each injection will sting for a few seconds to minimise the risk of sudden movement during the injection and dislodgement of the injection needle. After the procedure has been explained to the patient the primary lesion site or excision biopsy site is examined to determine the number of injections which will be required to produce an accurate result. The injections should surround the site of the melanoma and most patients will require 4 to 6 intradermal injections. Once the number of injections which will be needed has been determined, the patient should be told how many injections to expect (since without exception the patient will keep an accurate count of how many injections they receive!). Gloves should always be worn during the injection procedure. The test should not be performed after wide local excision as this disrupts the lymphatic drainage which renders the test unreliable.

The specific activity we use is 5 MBq in 0.05 ml and this is the preferred volume for each injection. A fine 25 gauge needle is used after the skin is cleaned with an alcohol wipe. With 99mTc antimony sulphide colloid there is usually pain at the site of injection. This can be quite intense, especially on the face, hands and feet. The most intense discomfort seems to occur with injections on the sole of the foot. When the injection is commenced a small bleb appears and the skin blanches at the site of injection, as a very high interstitial pressure is generated (Figure 4.1). Because of this it is very important that a gauze swab be placed over the needle before it is withdrawn from the skin, as failure to do so will result in both the injector and the skin around the injection site being sprayed with tracer and the patient's interstitial fluid. This is also a health hazard for the injector and is the reason that multidose injection vials should never be used for intradermal injections.[95] To avoid the needle being dislodged from the skin prematurely and avoid such contamination, it is worthwhile to have an assistant hold the hand or foot still during injection as it is a normal reflex to withdraw the limb from a source of pain. It is also advisable to place a large impervious incontinence sheet containing a cut-out window over the lesion site prior to injection to help avoid contamination of the surrounding skin of the patient, as this could confound later interpretation (as illustrated in Figure 4.1). Any swab used during tracer injection will become heavily contaminated with the tracer and should be discarded with the 'hot' waste and not with the normal garbage. The time of the commencement of intradermal injection should be noted, so that the rate of lymph flow can be determined accurately on the early dynamic scans.

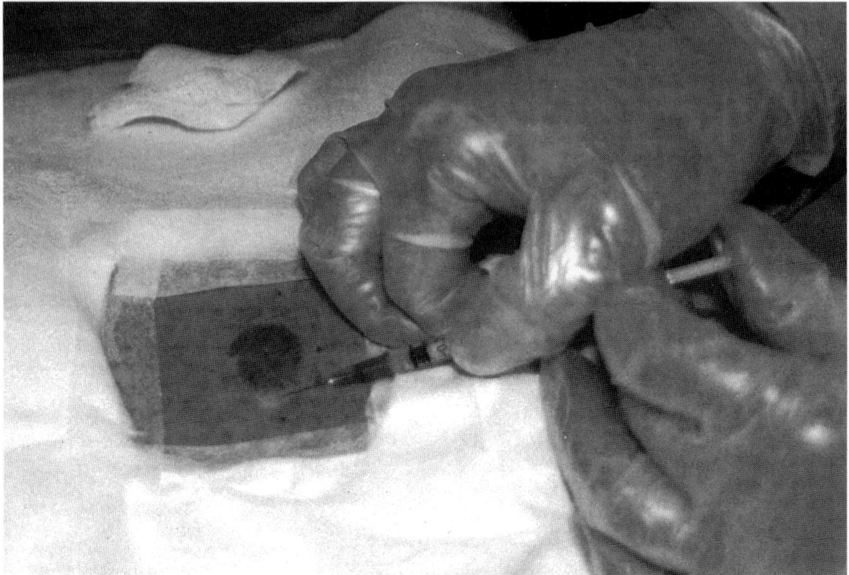

Figure 4.1 Intradermal injection of tracer

The interstitial pressure is quite high after intradermal injection of even small 0.1 ml injections. This causes the skin to blanche and a small bleb to form at the injection site. This high interstitial pressure may result in tracer being sprayed on the patient and the injector when the needle is removed unless a swab is placed over the needle before removing it from the skin.

4.3.2 Imaging the Patient

Injection of tracer should be completed as quickly as the situation allows and a dynamic acquisition commenced. Ten frames at 1 minute per frame is adequate to allow the rate of lymph flow to be measured in cm/min. This is a useful aid to the surgeon performing sentinel node surgery as it helps in timing the injection of blue dye prior to the induction of anaesthesia.[76] The early dynamic study is also an essential part of lymphoscintigraphy prior to sentinel node surgery, as it allows the confident identification of sentinel nodes as lymphatic channels drain directly to them (see Figure 3.8, pp. 42–3). The lymph channels should thus be followed until they reach the draining node field or fields. Lateral views of the head and neck and the axilla are often helpful at this stage to identify multiple sentinel nodes. Dynamic images are usually acquired for a total of 20 minutes.

Delayed scans are then performed 2½ hours after injection of tracer. These delayed scans should include all node fields which can possibly receive drainage from the injection site. Each static acquisition should be for 5–10 minutes to ensure that even very faint sentinel nodes are detected. Many workers use a transmission source to outline the patient during delayed imaging and we have incorporated this in our delayed imaging protocol. However, there are potential problems when using a transmission source. If the primary melanoma site is on a part of the skin from which drainage can be ambiguous, e.g. the trunk, head or neck, we strongly advise that during this delayed imaging phase a set of images be obtained without the transmission source in place. This is to ensure that all faint sentinel nodes in new node fields not suspected on dynamic imaging are found. Sometimes on the dynamic phase no lymph channel will be seen draining to a particular node field but on delayed scanning a faint but definite node will be seen. If this is in a new node field it is by definition a true sentinel node. Such faint nodes (Figure 4.2) are likely to be obscured by scattered radiation through the patient if a transmission source is used. A list of the recognised node fields which can directly drain the skin is listed in Table 4.2.

4.3.3 Expected Lymphatic Drainage Pathways

It should be emphasised that lymphatic drainage is unpredictable from any point on the skin. However, common patterns of drainage are present from various regions. In all areas drainage tends to be to ipsilateral node groups though contralateral drainage is not uncommon (Figure 4.3). A brief description of the common patterns follows.

Table 4.2 Node fields which directly drain lymph from the skin

Node fields
Axillary
Epitrochlear
Interpectoral
Para-vertebral
Retroperitoneal
Triangular intermuscular space
Right and left costal margin
Internal mammary
Groin
Popliteal
Cervical (Levels I–V)
Preauricular
Postauricular
Occipital
Supraclavicular

A

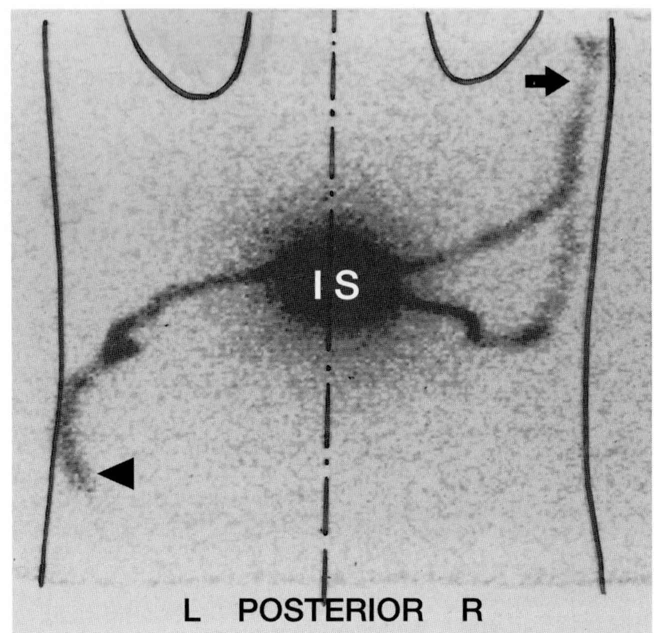

B

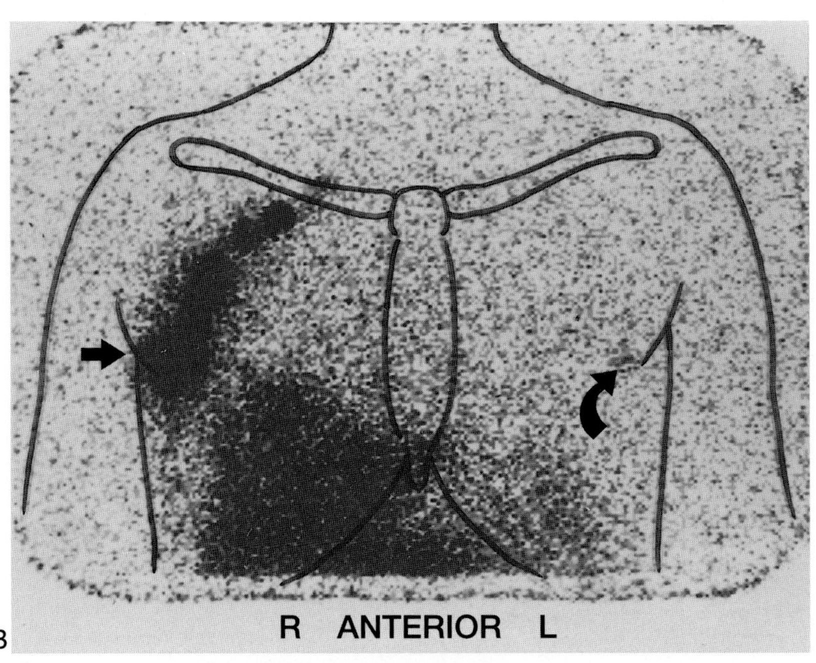

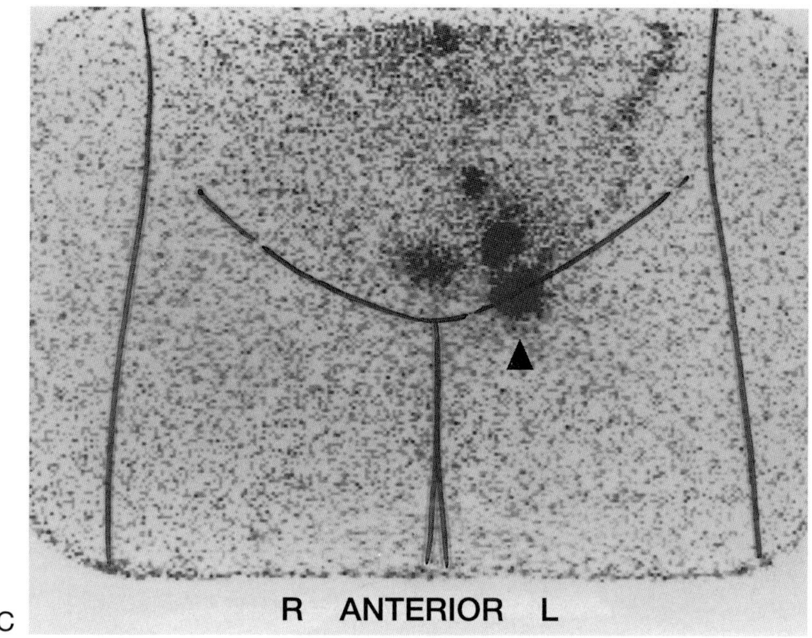

Figure 4.2 A transmission source may obscure faint sentinel nodes

The dynamic image (A) shows two dominant channels passing from the injection site (IS) on the mid back to the right axilla (arrow) and one channel passing towards the left groin (arrowhead). On delayed scans (B and C) bright nodes are seen in the right axilla (arrow) and the left groin (arrowhead) but there is also a faint sentinel node in the left axilla (curved arrow). Such a faint sentinel node is likely to have been obscured by scattered radiation through the patient if a transmission source is used to acquire these scans. Whenever such a situation is possible we always acquire two sets of delayed scans, one with and one without a transmission source, to avoid missing such faint sentinel nodes.

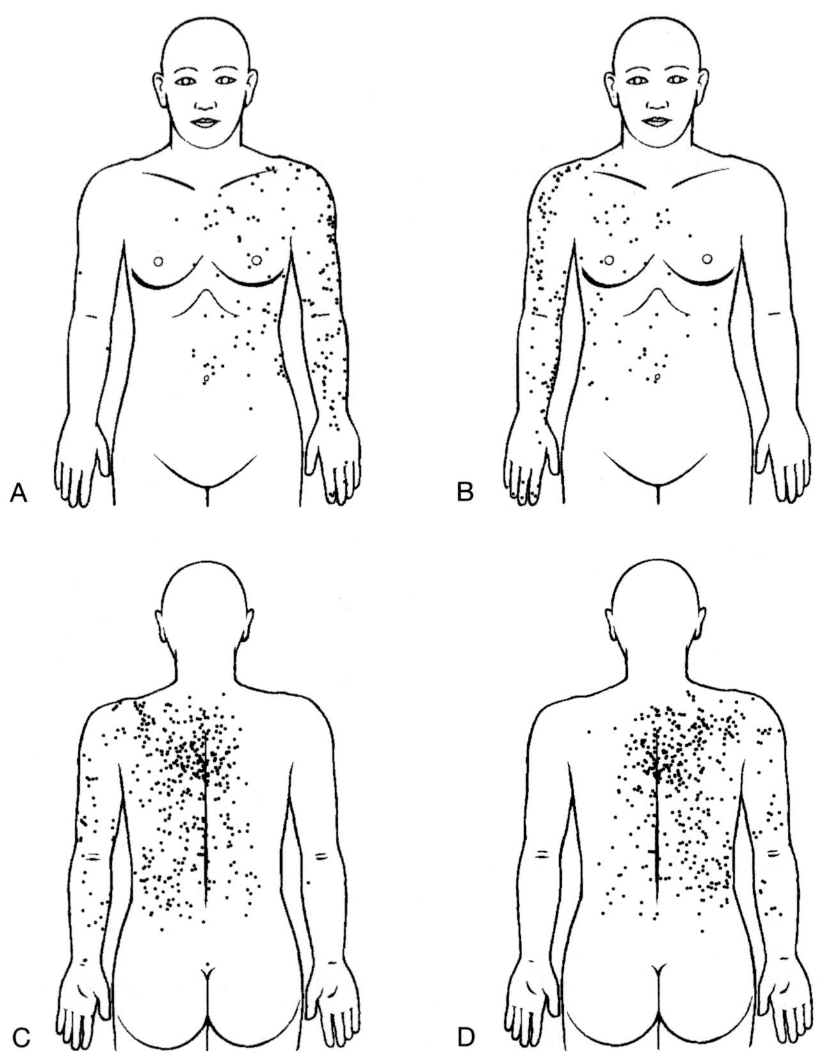

Figure 4.3 Sites on the trunk and arm which drain to the axilla

Anterior sites which drain to the left axilla (A), right axilla (B) and posterior sites which drain to the left axilla (C) and right axilla (D). The striking feature of sites draining to the right axilla and left axilla is the extent to which drainage can occur across the midline on the skin of the back. Melanoma sites can be quite lateral on the posterior trunk and still drain to the opposite axilla though this occurs almost without exception along with drainage to the ipsilateral axilla. Drainage across the midline to either axilla from the anterior trunk is less marked.

4.3.3.1 *Head and neck*

In the head and neck drainage from the anterior face and scalp tends to occur to parotid preauricular nodes and Level I to III cervical nodes. Drainage from the posterior scalp is generally to occipital, postauricular and Level V cervical nodes, while drainage from the skin of the neck is generally to Level I to V cervical nodes and supraclavicular nodes.

4.3.3.2 *Trunk*

Drainage from the anterior trunk is commonly to axillary (Figure 4.3), groin (Figure 4.4) and supraclavicular nodes (Figure 4.5), while drainage from the posterior trunk is generally to axillary (Figure 4.3), groin (Figure 4.4), and supraclavicular nodes (Figure 4.5). It is unusual for lymph drainage from the trunk not to include the axilla (Figure 4.6).

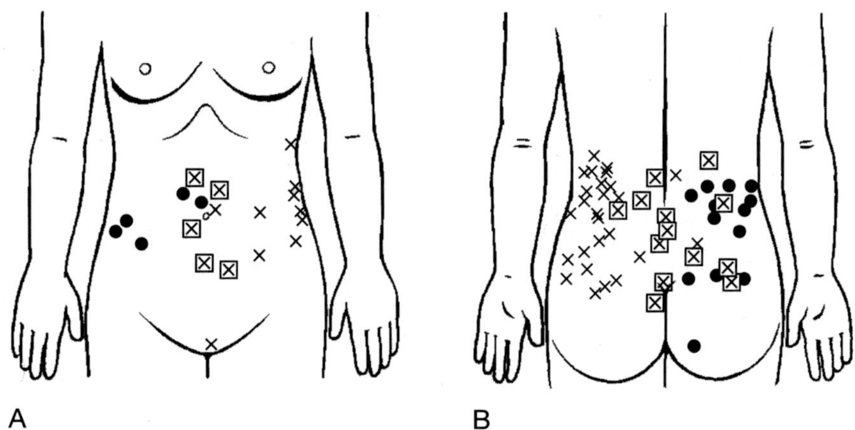

Figure 4.4 Truncal sites which drain to the groin nodes

A: Anterior torso sites which drain to the groin nodes. B: Posterior torso sites which drain to the groin. Circles indicate sites which drain to the right groin and crosses to the left groin. Boxed crosses drain to both groin node fields.

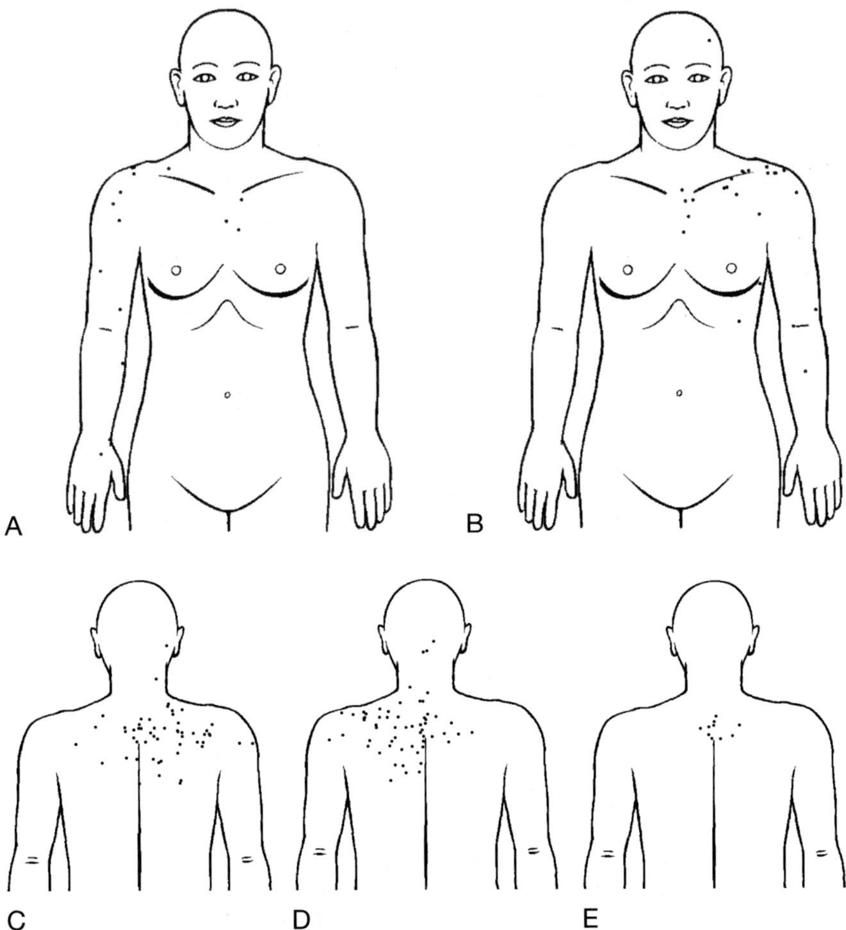

Figure 4.5 Drainage to the supraclavicular fossa

Anterior trunk sites which drained to the right supraclavicular fossa (A) and left supraclavicular fossa (B). There was only one site on the anterior trunk just above and to the left of the manubrium which showed drainage to the SCF bilaterally. Posterior trunk site which drained to the right SCF (C), the left SCF (D) and both the right and the left SCF (E). It is common for sites on the upper back to drain over the shoulders to the supraclavicular nodes as shown here. This can occur from quite well down the back sometimes from skin below the axilla. Drainage across the midline is not uncommon but drainage to both supraclavicular fossae occurs only from a small area of the skin in the midline below the base of the neck. Drainage to a supraclavicular fossa from the neck or head occurs sometimes though only some of these sites are shown here.

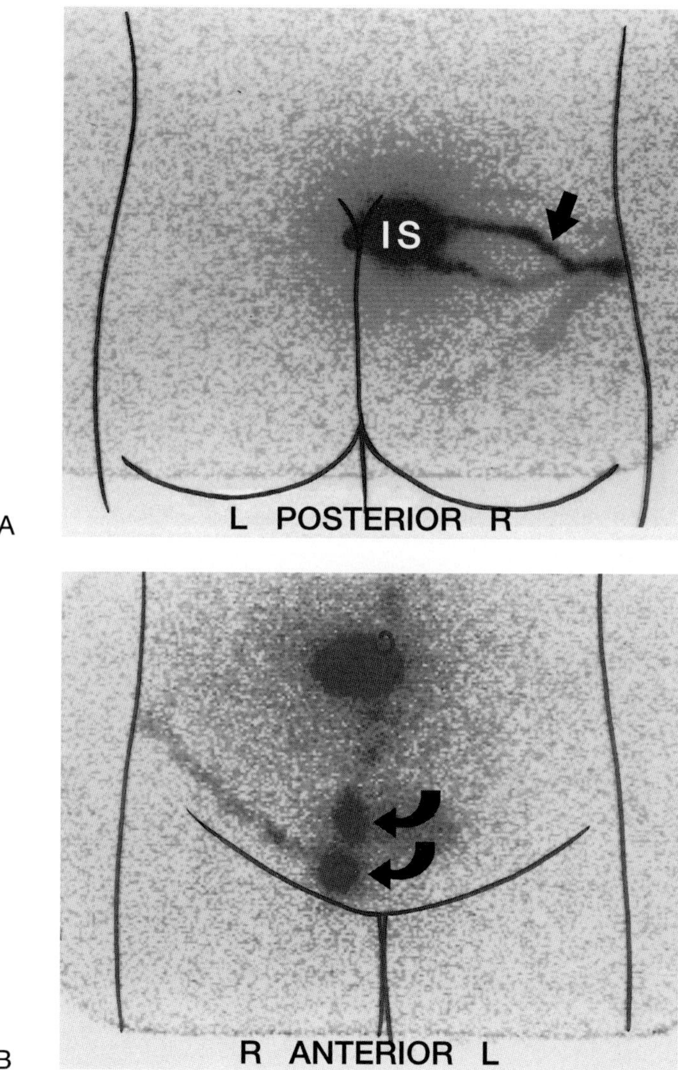

Figure 4.6 Lymph drainage from the trunk which does not include the axilla is unusual

A: This patient with an injection site (IS) just above and to the right of the natal cleft had drainage via 2 channels (arrow) to the right groin only on dynamic scan. B: On delayed imaging there were two sentinel nodes in the right groin (curved arrows), but in C (see page 62) no drainage whatsoever to either axilla. Most patients with primary sites on the trunk have drainage patterns which include some axillary drainage.

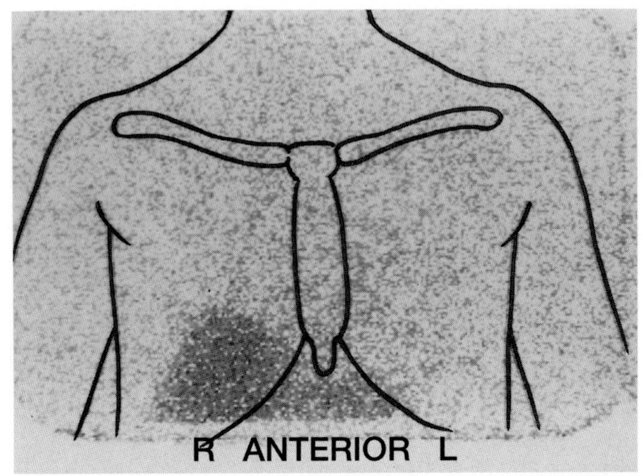

C

Figure 4.6 *Continued*

4.3.3.3 *Upper limb*

The usual drainage from the forearm is to the axilla with occasional drainage to epitrochlear nodes (Figure 4.7 and Figure 4.8), while drainage from the arm is usually to the axilla but with occasional drainage to supraclavicular nodes.

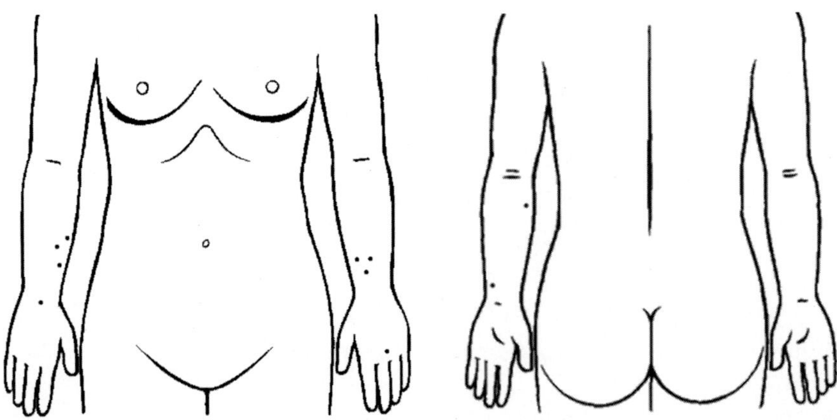

Figure 4.7 Sites which drain to the epitrochlear nodes

The sites which we have found draining to the epitrochlear node field are more widespread than has been described previously.

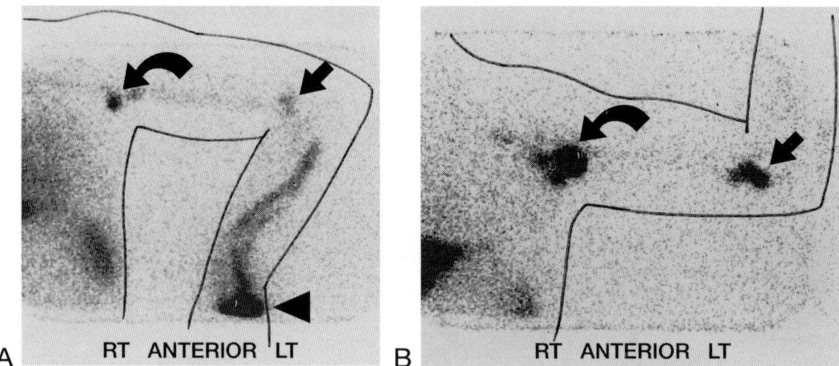

Figure 4.8 Drainage to sentinel nodes in the epitrochlear region

Dynamic phase (A) and delayed scan (B). Melanoma site on left wrist (arrowhead). This patient shows drainage to a sentinel node in the epitrochlear field (arrow), with a separate lymphatic channel passing to a sentinel node in the left axilla (curved arrow).

4.3.3.4 *Lower limb*

Drainage from the leg is to the groin with occasional drainage to popliteal nodes (Figure 4.9 and Figure 4.10) being seen, while drainage from the thigh is to groin nodes.

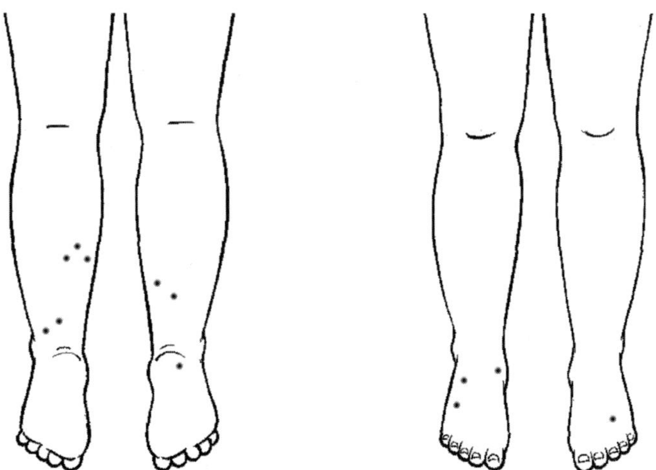

Figure 4.9 Sites which drain to the popliteal fossa

The sites which we have found draining to the popliteal fossa are spread over a wider distribution of the skin than others have found in the past.

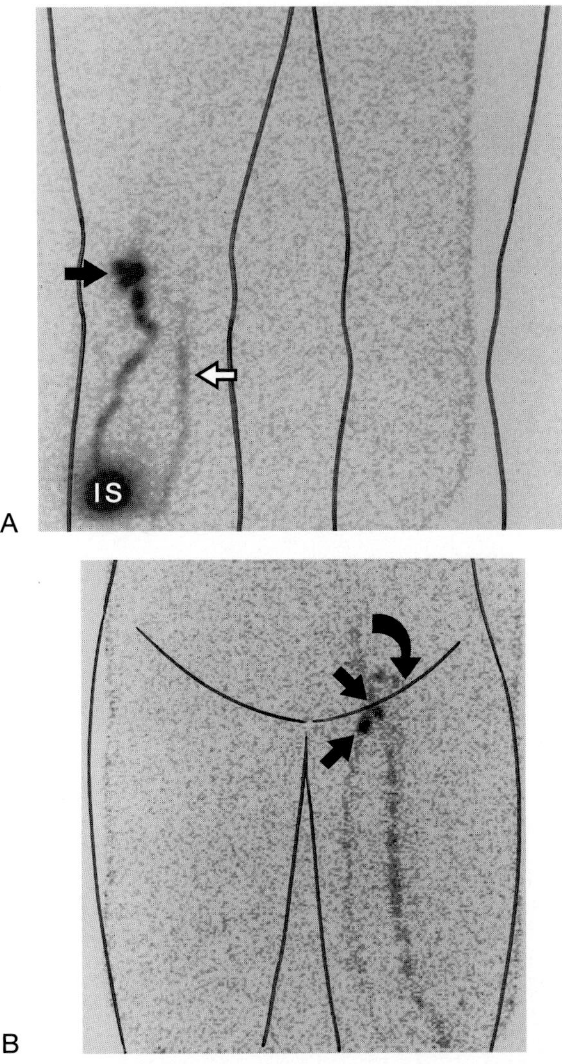

Figure 4.10 Drainage to sentinel nodes in the popliteal fossa

A: The dynamic study in the posterior projection over the legs shows tracer in the injection site (IS) on the posterior left calf and a channel passing to a sentinel node in the popliteal fossa (arrow) as well as tracer bypassing this area to drain directly to the groin (open arrow). B: Dynamic phase anteriorly over the groin shows 2 channels converging to reach 2 sentinel nodes in the groin (arrows). A third faint channel is seen passing to a node higher and laterally in the left groin (curved arrow). This is a channel which has passed on from the popliteal nodes upwards to the groin, thus this node is a second tier

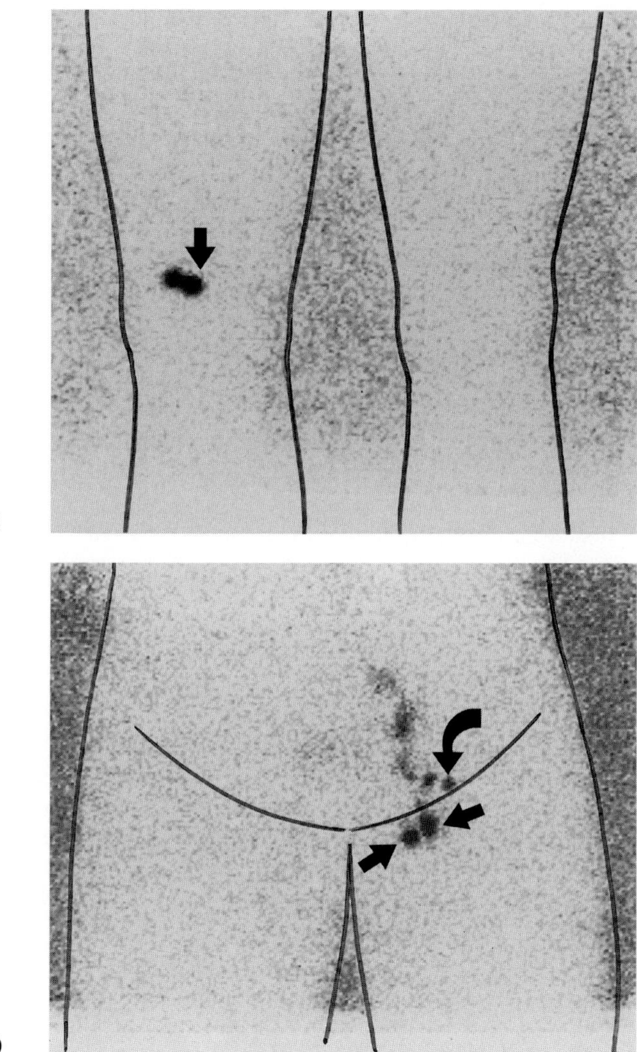

Figure 4.10 *Continued*

node as is the faint node medial to it. C: Delayed scan posteriorly over the popliteal fossa shows 2 sentinel nodes in the popliteal fossa (arrow). These nodes were very small at surgery measuring only 2–3 mm in length but both were blue stained and very ‘hot’ with the gamma probe. D: Delayed scan shows the 2 sentinel nodes in the groin (arrows) and fainter activity in several second tier nodes, including the node receiving second tier drainage from the popliteal fossa sentinel nodes (curved arrow).

4.3.4 Unusual Lymphatic Drainage Pathways

It is important to be aware of the possibility of unusual drainage patterns and to check whether non-standard node fields have received lymph drainage. These unusual drainage patterns include direct drainage to:

1. the triangular intermuscular space from the skin of the back;[96]
2. para-vertebral nodes from the loin posteriorly;[97, 98]
3. a right or left costal margin interval node and then on to internal mammary nodes from the periumbilical skin;[99]
4. supraclavicular fossa nodes from the forearm and wrist;[100]
5. interpectoral nodes from the forearm;[101]
6. postauricular nodes from the face and anterior scalp;[102]
7. Level 4 and 5 cervical nodes from the scalp;[102]
8. nodes across the midline especially on the back and the face;[97, 102]
9. occipital, parotid and Level 2 cervical nodes from the base of the neck;[102]
10. axillary nodes from the base of the neck;[102]
11. retroperitoneal nodes from the skin of the loin.[98]

Once all the appropriate node fields have been scanned, the sentinel nodes in each node field should be marked. The detail of this is described elsewhere,[103] but in summary it is done by marking the surface location of the node using a pinpoint tattoo of carbon black ink and a small cross of Castellani's paint (Figure 4.11). Marking must be performed with the patient in exactly the same position as that anticipated to be used during surgery. Failure to ensure this will mean that the skin mark will not overlay the node. The depth of the node beneath the skin can also be measured using an orthogonal view and by briefly imaging with a small radioactive point source placed on the skin at the site of the surface mark. The depth can then be measured electronically on the acquisition computer system or manually on the film.

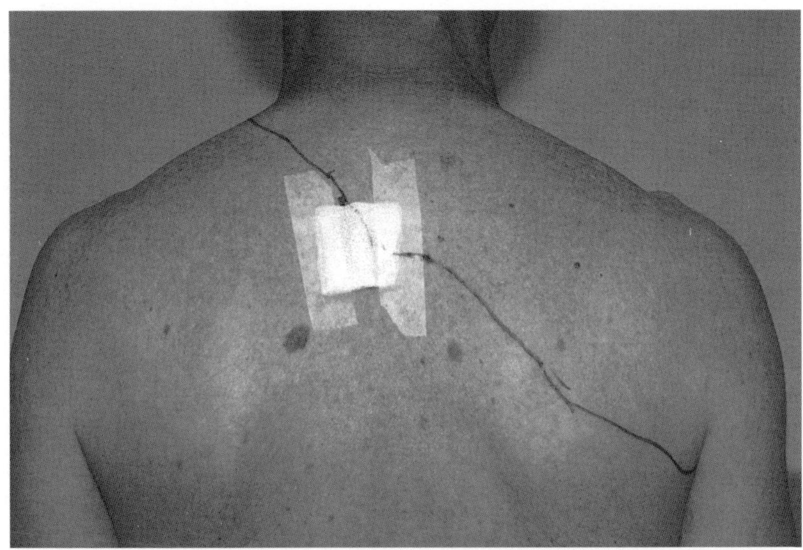

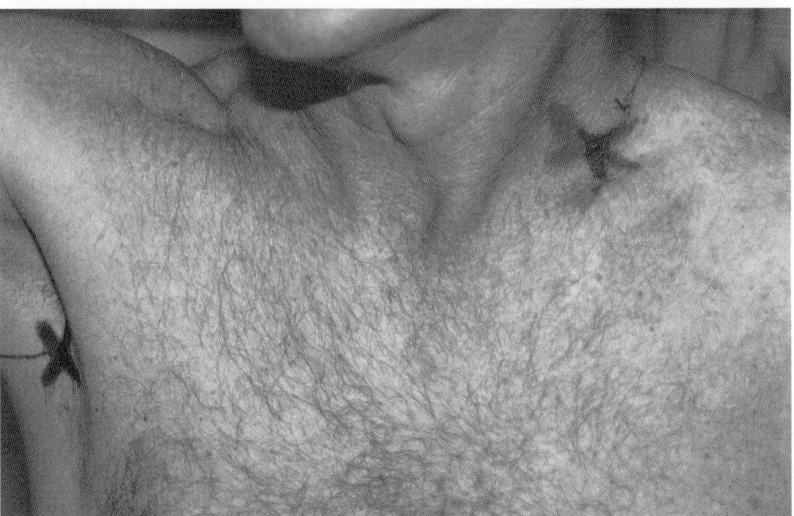

Figure 4.11 Marking the sentinel nodes during lymphoscintigraphy

This patient with an excision-biopsy site high on the back just to the left of midline showed a single dominant channel passing to the right axilla and a second channel passing over the left shoulder to the left supraclavicular fossa. The course of the lymphatic channel has been drawn on the skin and a single sentinel node in each node field point tattooed with carbon black ink and marked with a cross of Castellani's paint.

Chapter 5

THE SENTINEL LYMPH NODE CONCEPT IN MELANOMA

5.1 DEFINITION OF A SENTINEL NODE

A sentinel node was defined by Morton and colleagues as 'the first lymph node to receive drainage from a lesion site'.[104] This definition is open to misinterpretation especially if there is more than one sentinel node. We prefer the definition, 'any lymph node receiving direct lymphatic drainage from a lesion site'[103] as this essentially describes the physiology of the sentinel node concept itself and includes all possible scenarios including multiple sentinel nodes and interval nodes (Figure 5.1).

5.2 INTERVAL NODES

Interval nodes are lymph nodes draining a lesion site which lie between that lesion site and a recognised node field. They receive lymphatic drainage directly from the lesion site and all interval nodes are therefore, by definition, sentinel nodes (Figure 5.2), unless they receive tracer which has previously passed through another interval node. This phenomenon occurs when several interval nodes lie along the path of a single lymphatic vessel.

5.3 SENTINEL NODES

The term 'sentinel' lymph nodes was first used in the medical literature to refer to the nodes in the deep inferior cervical group into which the subclavian lymphatic trunks sometimes drained just before they joined the thoracic duct or right lymphatic duct. These nodes were therefore the last possible lymph node filter before the lymph fluid contents entered the venous circulation at the confluence of the internal jugular and subclavian veins. The nodes were thus the final 'sentinel' for the entry of metastases into the circulation.[66]

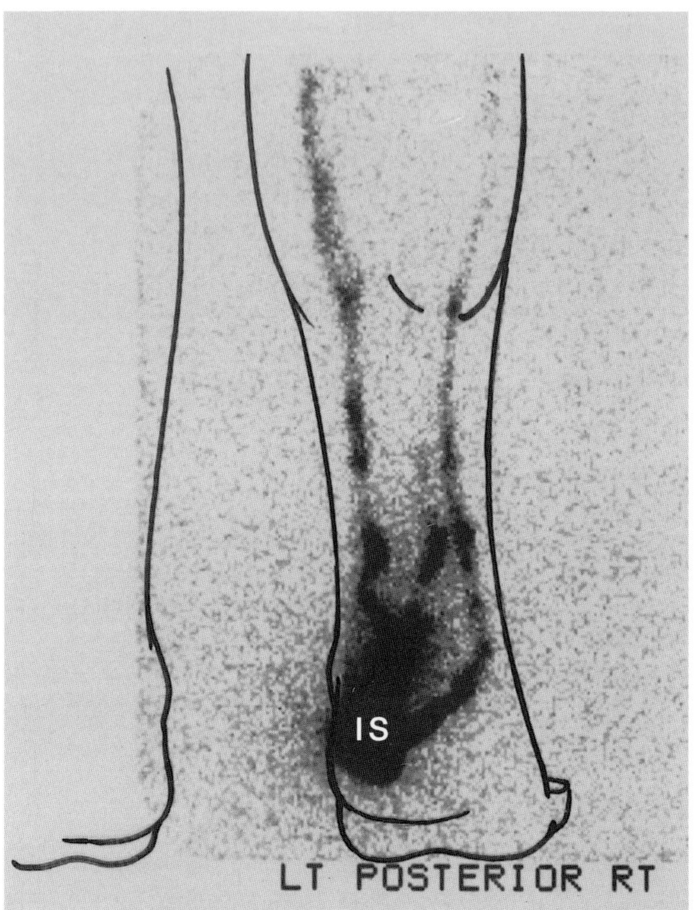

Figure 5.1 Multiple sentinel nodes are common in the groin with leg injections

A: Multiple channels are seen passing upwards from the injection site (IS) just above the right heel medially. B: In the upper thigh the lymph channels are seen to diverge to meet multiple sentinel nodes (arrows). There is also a very tortuous channel which doubles back on itself in the thigh before finding its way to a small faint sentinel node high in the right groin (curved arrow). It would be impossible to identify this small sentinel node which contains very little radioactivity without high quality lymphoscintigraphy.

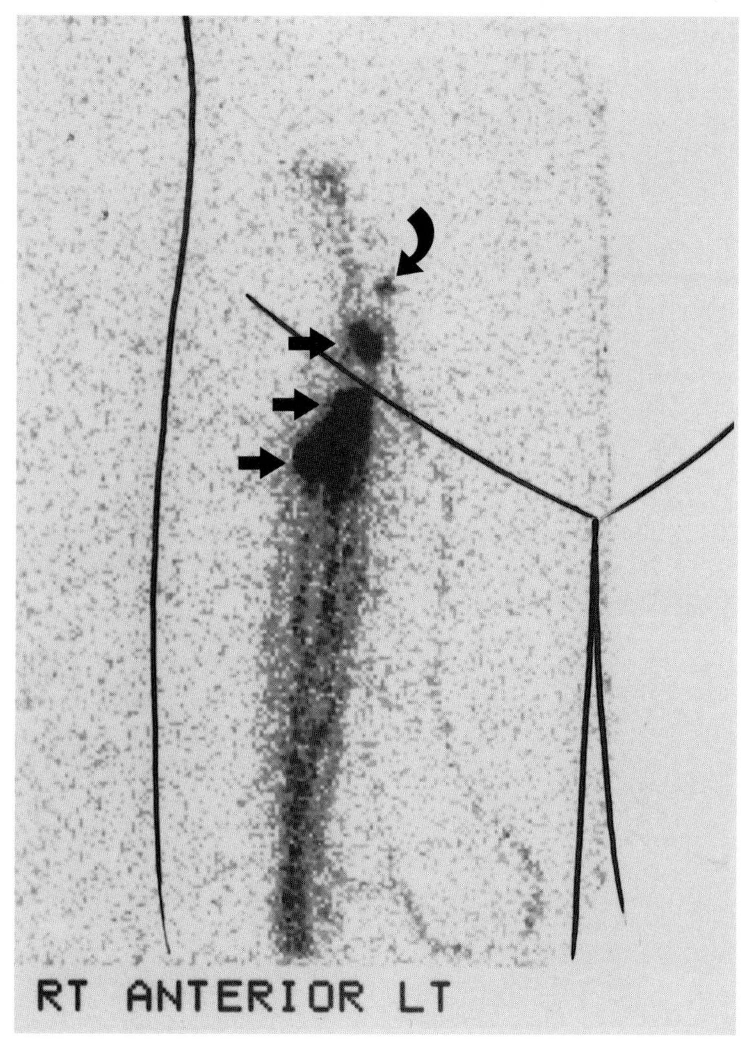

B

Figure 5.1 *Continued*

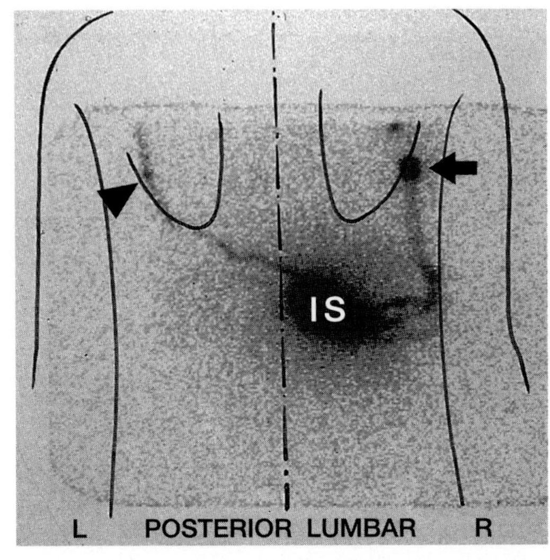

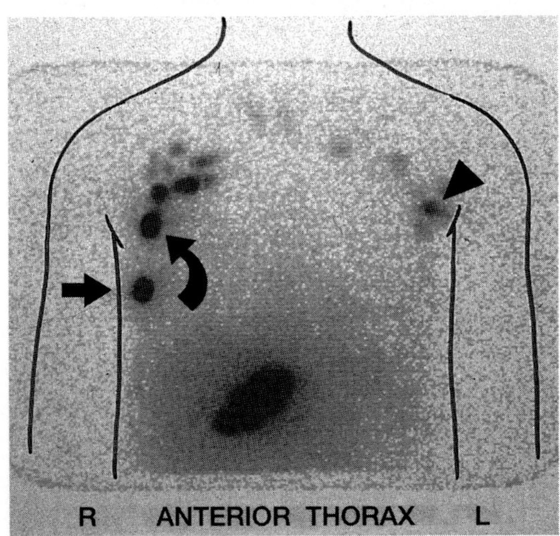

Figure 5.2 Interval node in mid axillary line

The early dynamic image (A) in the posterior view shows several channels passing from the injection site (IS) on the mid back to the right of midline towards the right axilla, with one of the channels meeting an interval node in the mid axillary line (arrow). A single channel is also seen crossing the midline towards the left axilla (arrowhead). The delayed scan (B) in the anterior view shows the interval node (arrow), the sentinel node in the left axilla (arrowhead) and sentinel nodes in the right axilla (curved arrow). Interval nodes in the mid axillary line are not uncommon in patients with primary sites on the mid back towards the loin.

The term 'sentinel' nodes was also used by Cabanas to describe the lymph nodes which usually drained the penis.[105] He proposed that these nodes, which lay in the superficial inguinal area associated with the superficial epigastric vein, would be the ones to harbour metastases if any were present in lymph nodes. He described good survival if these nodes were excised and were negative for metastases on histology. Others found a significant false negative rate with recurrence occurring in other 'non-sentinel' nodes during follow-up.[106, 107] All of these studies involved a standard dissection of the medial group of superficial inguinal nodes and no dye or radiotracer was used. There was also no intraoperative method employed to locate draining nodes. This is analogous to calling the axillary nodes the 'sentinel' nodes for patients with melanoma on the forearm.

Neither of the above references to 'sentinel' nodes is relevant to the concept of the sentinel node as later defined by Morton and colleagues.[104] The sentinel node is the individual node or nodes which receive the lymph draining directly from the tumour site. Morton was the first to make this distinction clear, and this is the concept of the sentinel node as used and accepted in the medical literature today. This distinction also leads to a completely different surgical approach from that taken by Cabanas.

There is usually only one sentinel node in node fields which drain the skin of the trunk though there may be multiple node fields draining certain parts of the skin of the trunk. The axilla and groin both average 1.3 sentinel nodes when drainage occurs from the skin of the trunk.

Multiple sentinel nodes are more likely to occur in the groin (Figure 5.1) with lower limb lesion sites and in the cervical, occipital, preauricular and postauricular node fields with lesion sites on the head and neck. From the upper thigh there is frequently a bifurcation of the lymphatic channels so that multiple sentinel nodes are seen in the groin, even when only one or two dominant channels drain the lesion site on the early dynamic images. With lesion sites on the lower limb there are on average 3.3 sentinel nodes in the groin. For the head and neck there are on average 2.7 sentinel nodes per patient and 85% of patients have multiple sentinel nodes.

These multiple sentinel nodes in individual node fields reflect the varying physiology of the lymphatic system in different parts of the body, and are not an artefact caused by the use of a particular colloid. If multiple sentinel nodes are not being found in the groin with leg injections in a significant number of patients this indicates poor mapping of the lymphatic system by the radiocolloid being used. It is a fallacious argument to claim preference for a large particle colloid because 'it shows only the one sentinel node', as this simply means that other true sentinel nodes are being missed. For the sentinel node biopsy method to be reliable, all sentinel nodes must be found and removed, not just a convenient one or two hot nodes found with large particle colloids. Some researchers appear to be losing focus in their search for the sentinel node. They appear to be concentrating on removing one or two 'hot' nodes rather than seeking to accurately map the pattern of lymphatic drainage from the primary site and then locating and excising the sentinel nodes which will almost always be the 'hottest' nodes in the node field. It needs to be remembered however that less 'hot' second tier nodes will sometimes remain behind in the node field after a successful sentinel node biopsy. Alternatively on occasions a sentinel node will have only a small amount of tracer compared to other sentinel nodes in the field and such complex situations need high quality lymphoscitigraphy to resolve (Figure 5.1). They can not be accurately resolved using a gamma probe alone.

Sentinel nodes are found by following the lymphatic channels on dynamic lymphoscintigraphy and identifying each node which actually receives a channel directly (Figure 5.1). Sometimes, because of the resolution limitations of lymphoscintigraphy, it will be impossible to tell whether a particular lymph channel bypasses one sentinel node to reach a higher node. This is most frequently a problem in the groin, following injections in the leg. Under these circumstances the situation will need to be checked at the time of surgery by identifying and tracing blue-stained lymphatics after injecting blue dye at the primary tumour site. During surgery whenever possible the sentinel node is confirmed as the node receiving the blue lymphatic channel and staining blue. A gamma detection probe can also be used during surgery to confirm that the sentinel node thus found is 'hot' and that the residual node field counts are low after it has been removed.

In some patients no dominant lymph channel will be seen draining to a particular node field on the dynamic images, however a node will be seen in that node field on delayed images. Even though this node may be very faint it must nevertheless be a sentinel node and therefore should be removed during the biopsy procedure (Figure 5.3).

5.4 DISTINGUISHING SENTINEL NODES FROM SECOND TIER LYMPH NODES

A second tier lymph node is any node which receives lymph flow which has previously passed through the filter function of a sentinel node.

As mentioned previously, there is a variable incidence of tracer movement onward from the sentinel nodes to second tier nodes. This correlates directly with the speed of lymph flow from a particular skin region.[86] High lymph flow is associated with an increased incidence of activity in second tier nodes. Thus second tier nodes are more common in the groin than elsewhere, since higher lymph flow rates are more common in lymph channels draining the leg. However, high flow rates are occasionally seen in other parts of the body, thus

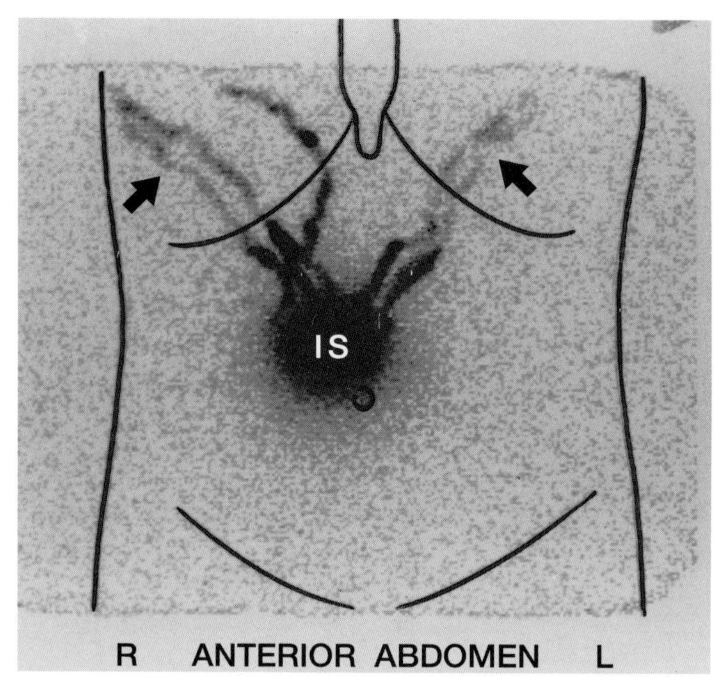

A

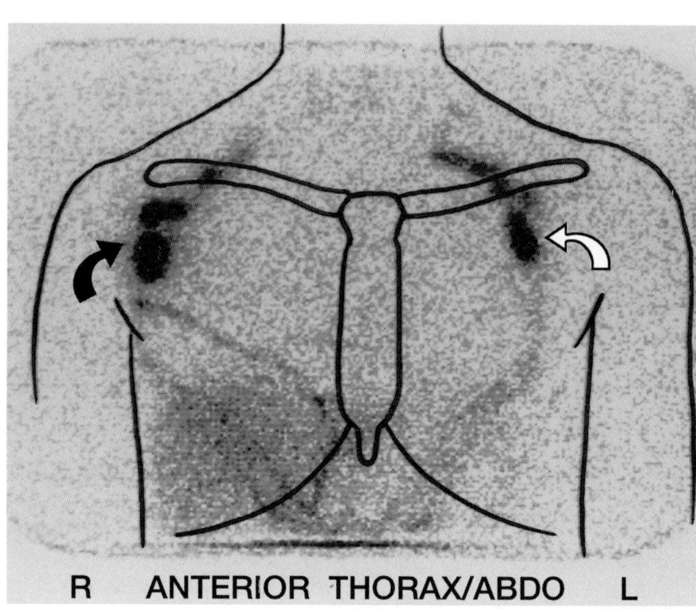

B

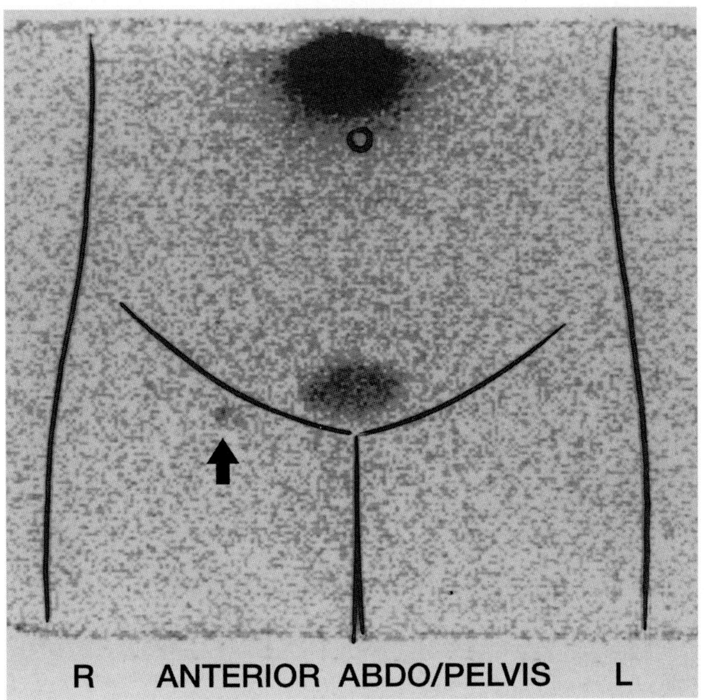

Figure 5.3 A sentinel node may only be detected on delayed imaging

The dynamic scan (A) shows multiple channels (diagonal arrows) passing from the injection site (IS) just above and to the right of the umbilicus. The delayed scans (B and C) show activity in multiple sentinel nodes in the right axilla (curved arrow) and left axilla (open curved arrow). Faint activity however is also present in a single sentinel node in the right groin (vertical arrow). Though no channel was seen passing to the right groin on the dynamic scan there is no doubt that this is a sentinel node in the right groin, which must be removed for the sentinel node biopsy method to be successful in this patient. Such a node which is seen only on two hour delayed imaging will not be detected if a gamma probe alone is used 20–30 minutes following injection of radiocolloid, and probably would not be visualised at all if large particle colloids were used in this patient.

obvious second tier activity can sometimes be seen in the axilla as well as the groin (Figure 5.4). Several features are important in helping to distinguish sentinel nodes from second tier nodes. If a lymph channel can be seen passing directly to a node from the injection site during the dynamic phase of lymphoscintigraphy, that is clearly a sentinel node regardless of the amount of tracer which migrates to the node, i.e. sentinel nodes vary in the intensity of tracer uptake and occasionally sentinel nodes will be 'colder' than second tier nodes in the same node field (Figure 5.1).

Sometimes no movement of tracer is seen on the dynamic image and activity in a particular node field is only evident on delayed imaging (Figure 5.3). In this situation other methods are needed to identify second tier nodes.

Second tier nodes tend to be more central in the same node field or lie in a node field which is more central on the lymphatic pathway to the thoracic duct, e.g. a sentinel node in the femoral area may have a second tier node seen higher in the femoral area or in the inguinal node field and a sentinel node in the inguinal area may have a second tier node in the iliac or obturator area.

Any node seen on delayed scans which is more peripheral to a sentinel node seen on dynamic imaging must be considered as another sentinel node and marked as such. Likewise a node which is seen only on delayed imaging but which lies lateral to or medial to a known sentinel node, e.g. in the groin must be considered another sentinel node (Figure 5.5) unless a channel can be seen passing onwards from the sentinel node to the other node (Figure 5.6).

Occasionally 2 lymphatic channels will appear to reach a single sentinel node in the groin but at about the same time tracer is seen passing beyond this node to a second node higher in the groin. In this situation both nodes must be marked and the true status of the higher node checked at the time of surgery. If a separate blue channel is seen bypassing the first node and passing directly to the higher node, then by definition this is a second sentinel node. Sometimes, as mentioned in section 1.2.2., the anatomic arrangement of the afferent lymphatic vessel and the lymph node means that the lymph is only partially subjected to the filter function of the node and some of the lymph fluid will pass unfiltered on to the next node.[24] This will be seen on lymphoscintigraphy as the rapid appearance of a second node more centrally in the node field after an apparent single channel has entered a sentinel node. When this is seen on lymphoscintigraphy the second node must also be marked as a potential second sentinel node. The resolution limitations of lymphoscintigraphy mean that these situations can only be confirmed at operation. As a general rule second tier nodes have less activity than sentinel nodes but this is not universally the case (Figure 5.1).

Using all of the above techniques it will be unusual for a second tier node to be mistaken for a sentinel node.

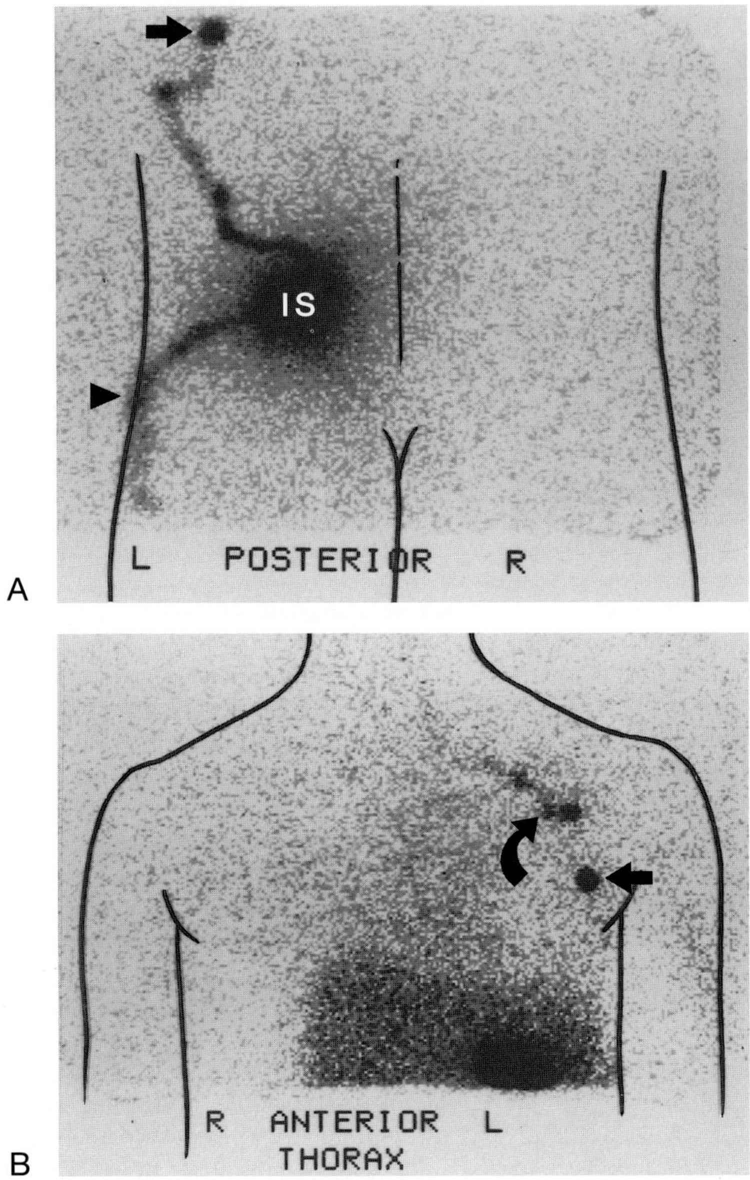

Figure 5.4 Obvious second tier nodes

The dynamic scan (A) shows a single dominant channel passing to a single sentinel node in the left axilla (arrow) from the injection site (IS) on the low back to the left of midline. A single dominant channel is also seen passing around the left side anteriorly to the left groin (arrowhead).

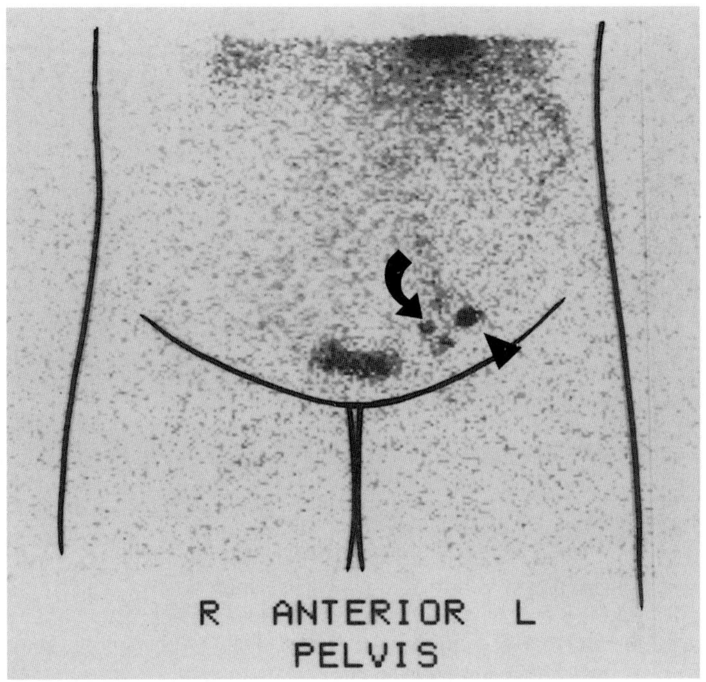

Figure 5.4 *Continued*

On the delayed scans (B and C) activity is seen in the single sentinel node in the left axilla (arrow), and the left groin (arrowhead), however obvious activity is seen in second tier nodes in both the axilla and groin (curved arrows). This phenomenon relates directly to the speed of lymph flow from the injection site and is thus more common in the groin with leg injections than elsewhere on the body.

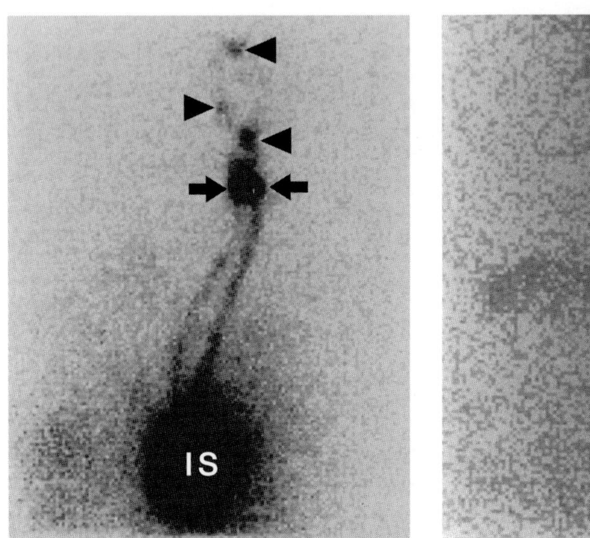

A

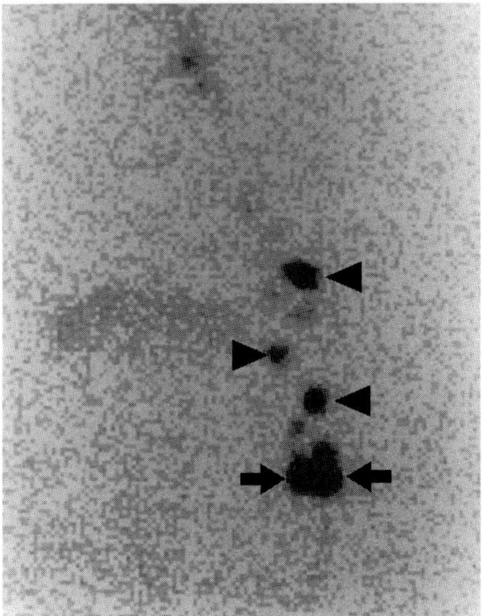

B

Figure 5.5 Differentiating sentinel nodes from second tier nodes

Nodes which lie medial or lateral to a known sentinel node but which appear only on delayed imaging should be considered as probable separate sentinel nodes unless proven otherwise at surgery. A: In this study 2 early channels were present passing upwards from the injection site in the left thigh (IS) to the left groin where they met 2 sentinel nodes in the femoral area (arrows). These 2 nodes are often the sentinel nodes in the groin and they lie anterior to and on each side of the femoral vein. Activity promptly passes on to 3 second tier nodes (arrowheads). B: The delayed scan over the groin shows similar findings and reveals that the second tier nodes in the groin can sometimes be quite 'hot'. As mentioned previously this phenomenon is related to the speed of lymph flow through the lymph channels. If no flow is seen in early images and one is faced with a delayed image, such as in B, all 5 hot nodes should be marked as potential sentinel nodes and the situation checked at surgery after blue dye injection. Nodes lying side by side such as the 2 femoral nodes (arrows) are almost always both sentinel nodes but nodes higher or more centrally placed in the node field (arrowheads) are usually second tier nodes.

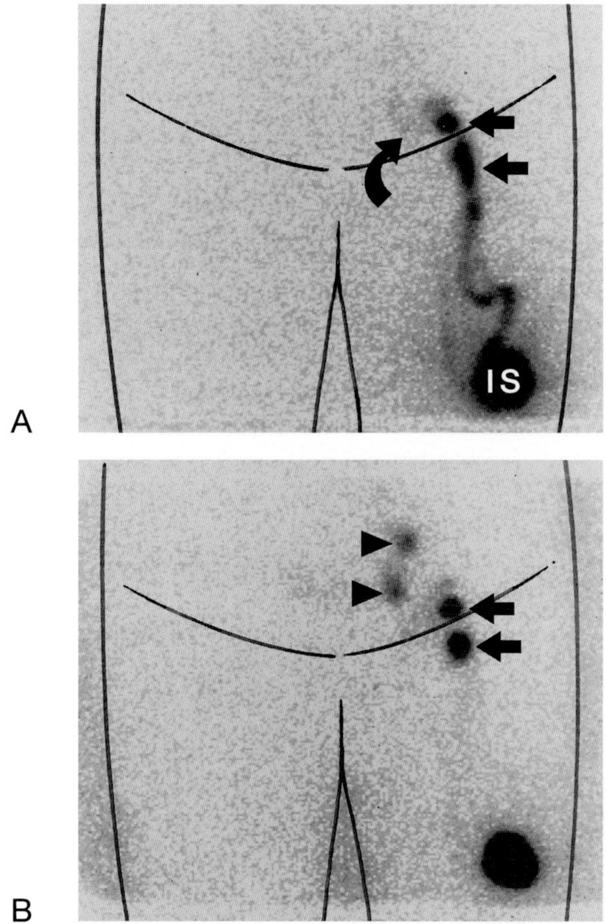

Figure 5.6 Tortuous channels can be checked at surgery

A: This dynamic study shows tracer in the injection site (IS) on the left thigh and several channels converging on 2 sentinel nodes in the left groin (arrows). There is an 'S' shaped lymph channel (curved arrow) doubling back upon itself to reach a second tier node in the left groin some distance medial to the higher of the 2 sentinel nodes. B: The delayed scan shows tracer in the 2 sentinel nodes (arrows) and tracer in 2 second tier nodes (arrowheads). The lower of the 2 second tier nodes is placed some distance medial to the 2 sentinel nodes. This node was marked as a possible sentinel node and the situation was checked at surgery. An 'S' shaped channel was found passing onwards from the higher of the 2 sentinel nodes to the medial node thus confirming its status as a second tier node. This is an unusual case and most nodes which lie some distance medial or lateral to a sentinel node in the groin are themselves separate sentinel nodes.

5.5 DRAINAGE TO MULTIPLE NODE FIELDS

Multiple node fields draining a single skin site are common on the trunk and also for lesion sites around the base of the neck and around the midline of the body, both anteriorly and posteriorly. The skin sites which drain to 2 or more node fields tend to be congregated around the midline of the trunk, in a band around the waist, across the shoulders posteriorly and in the head and neck region (Figure 5.7). Drainage to 3 node fields is seen in a similar distribution over the posterior trunk and in the periumbilical area anteriorly as well as the head and neck (Figure 5.8), but drainage to 4 or more node fields is seen only occasionally in the head and neck and from very restricted areas of the trunk. These truncal areas lie between the scapulae and at around L2 level near the midline on the back (where Sappey's lines cross) and in the periumbilical area on the anterior trunk (Figure 5.9).

5.6 LOCATING AND MARKING THE SENTINEL NODES

The concept of using the sentinel node as a marker for the presence or absence of metastatic disease in a regional node field was first proposed by Morton et al. in 1992.[104] They injected blue dye intradermally prior to surgery and then surgically traced the lymphatic channels until the sentinel node in the draining node field was reached. This procedure was technically difficult, and surgeons needed a learning period involving about 50 operations before they were capable of accurately performing the procedure. The study did show, however, that if the sentinel node was confidently identified as being blue stained, with a blue afferent lymphatic channel entering it, then it provided a reliable assessment of that node field with an accuracy of 99%. This meant that if the sentinel node was negative for metastases then the other lymph nodes in that node field would also be negative for metastases.

Subsequently others have successfully used a gamma probe at surgery immediately following injection of 99mTc sulphur colloid intradermally around the lesion site in melanoma patients. Krag et al. in 1995 reported successful location of the sentinel node in 98% of 121 patients.[108] The gamma probe method had the advantage of simplicity over Morton's surgical dissection method and was more easily taught to other surgeons who were interested in applying the technique.

We had been performing lymphoscintigraphy in patients with melanoma on the trunk to determine the location of the draining node fields for some years by this time[97] and we saw no reason why we could not use our lymphoscintigram technique to locate the sentinel node. By modifying the scanning method we were able to show that the sentinel node could be accurately located using lymphoscintigraphy prior to surgery.[103]

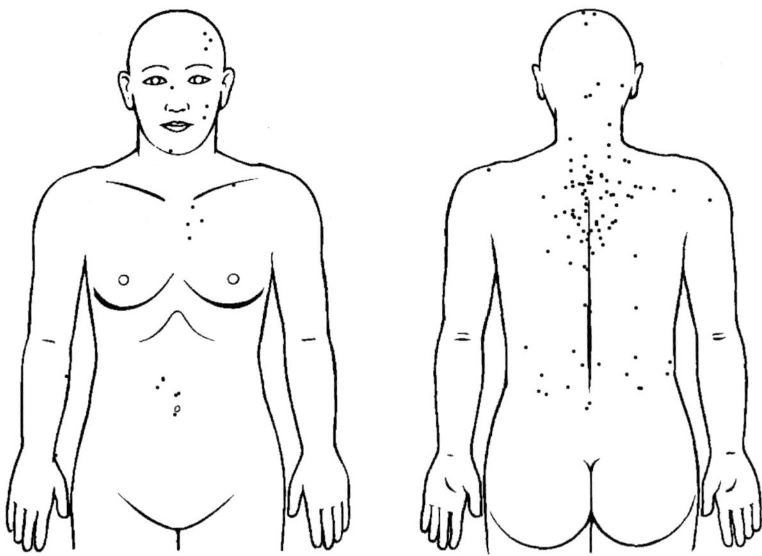

Figure 5.7 Sites showing drainage to two or more node fields

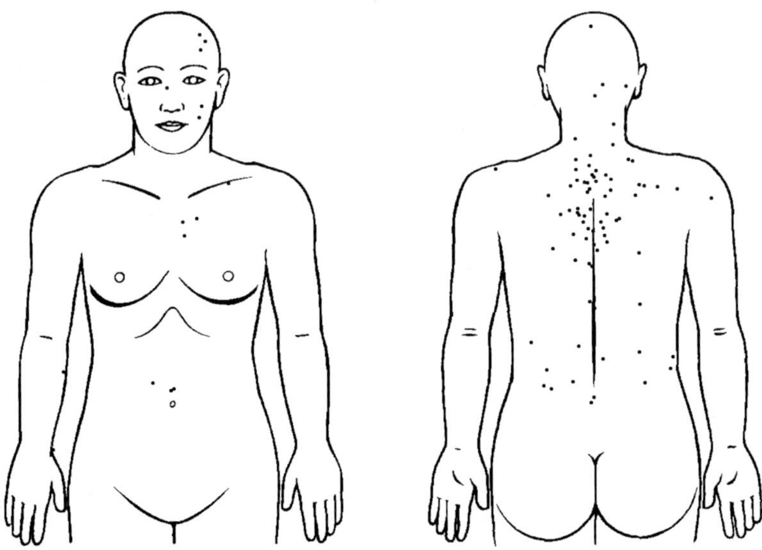

Figure 5.8 Sites showing drainage to three node fields

Drainage to 3 node fields occurs from sites over a wide area of the back especially at waist level and higher on the back towards the midline. The head and neck is also a site where drainage to multiple node fields is common.

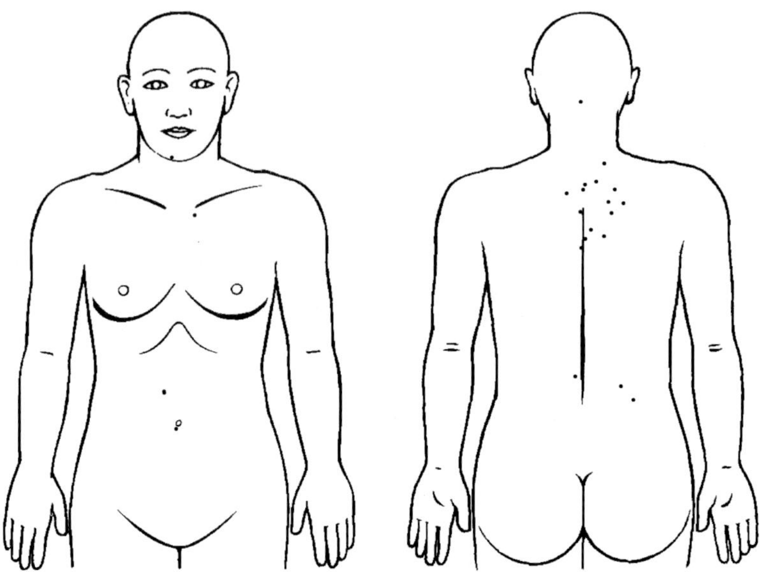

Figure 5.9 Sites showing drainage to four node fields

Drainage to 4 node fields occurs from a very restricted area of the back between the scapulae and also at about the L2 level close to the midline which is in the region of the intersection of Sappey's original lines of demarcation on the back.

We now routinely mark the surface location of the sentinel node or nodes (see Figure 4.11) and also measure the depth of the node beneath the skin mark in the anticipated position to be used for surgery, so that the surgeon can make a small incision over the mark and in most patients rapidly locate the node. Blue dye is injected just prior to the surgical exploration (Figure 5.10) and the patient exercises the relevant body part to encourage rapid movement of the blue dye via the lymphatic channels. This should be done before the patient is anaesthetised since much slower migration of the dye will occur after the patient is anaesthetised and placed on the operating table. The surgeon then makes an incision at the site marked on the skin during lymphoscintigraphy and cuts down to the depth indicated on the scan (Figure 5.11). He/she then finds the sentinel node as a blue staining node with a blue stained lymph channel entering it.

We also find the gamma probe is very useful in locating the sentinel node if

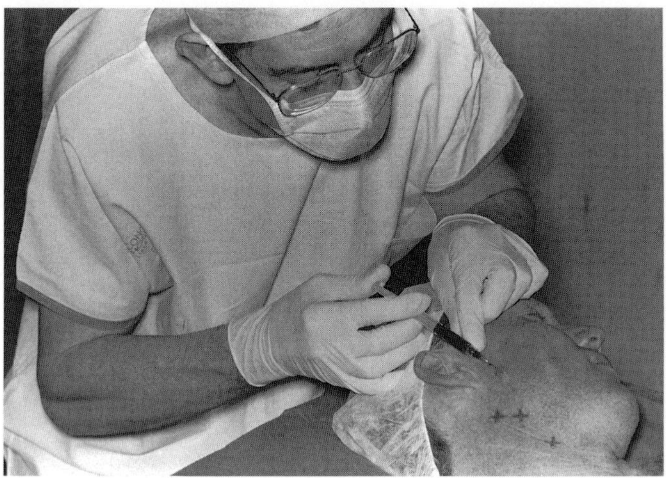

Figure 5.10 Preoperative injection of blue dye

The surgeon injects blue dye around the excision biopsy site anterior to the right ear just before surgery. Crosses which mark the location of 3 sentinel nodes in this patient can be seen in the right upper neck. The injection site is then massaged and when possible the patient exercises the body part prior to the induction of anaesthesia.

surgery is done within 24 hours of the lymphoscintigram. The sentinel node will still usually be the most radioactive lymph node in the node field and even at 24 hours is often the only radioactive node. This is true especially in the axilla. The gamma probe is particularly useful in obese patients who can have large amounts of adipose tissue in the axilla; in some patients this will mean that the sentinel node is 8 to 10 cm beneath the skin mark made at lymphoscintigraphy. In such patients the gamma probe greatly speeds up the location of the sentinel node and it is useful even in the slim axilla to ensure that the surgical search is headed in the right direction (Figure 5.12). The sentinel node can be recognised as the node containing the high count rate and complete removal of the sentinel node can be confirmed by documenting a fall in the residual count rate in the node field after removal of the sentinel node. We believe that the best method of accurately locating the sentinel lymph nodes is by using a combination of these techniques and others have also found this to be true.[109]

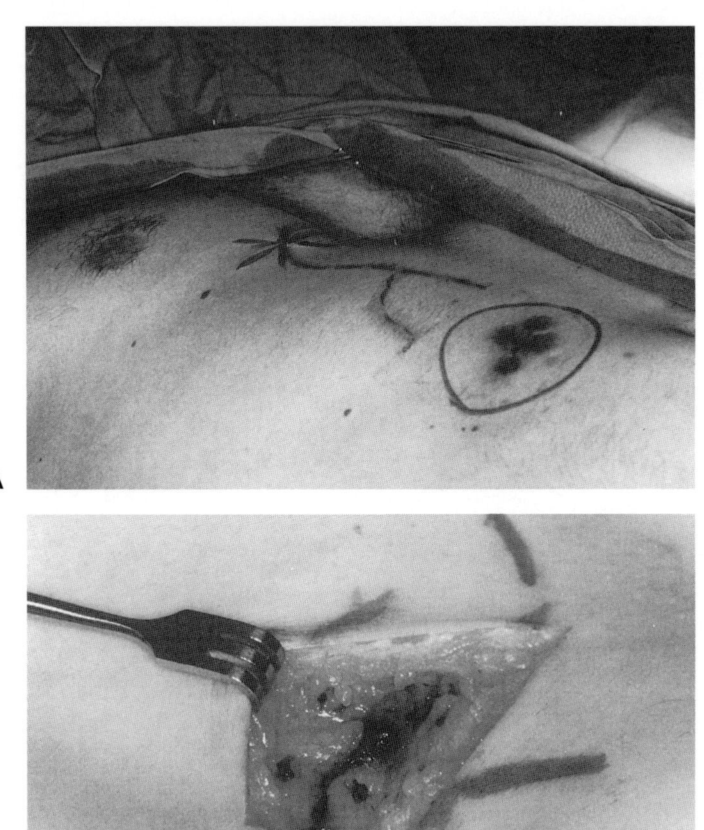

Figure 5.11 Locating the blue staining sentinel node

A: The lymphatic channel passing from the periumbilical excision site to a right costal margin sentinel node has been marked on the skin and the sentinel node marked with a cross. Four injections of blue dye are seen around the primary site (circled) and an incision has been made exactly at the cross marked on the skin over the right costal margin. B: Retractors pull the skin back to reveal the blue stained channel passing into the blue staining sentinel lymph node immediately beneath the cross marked on the skin.

5.7 THE SYDNEY MELANOMA UNIT METHOD OF SENTINEL NODE BIOPSY IN MELANOMA

At the Sydney Melanoma Unit we routinely use *preoperative lymphoscintigraphy* the day before surgery to map lymphatic drainage. This allows any unusual drainage patterns to be identified and anticipated at the time of surgery. The speed of lymphatic transport of the colloid is recorded. The draining node fields are identified and all interval nodes and sentinel nodes are located and marked on the skin. This is done even if drainage to a particular sentinel node is very slow or if it has only a small amount of radioactivity. Prior to the induction of anaesthesia, *blue dye* is injected intradermally around the lesion or excision biopsy site. The timing of this injection is determined by the speed of lymph flow observed during lymphoscintigraphy. If flow is slow, the dye is injected earlier and the patient is encouraged to quite vigorously exercise the

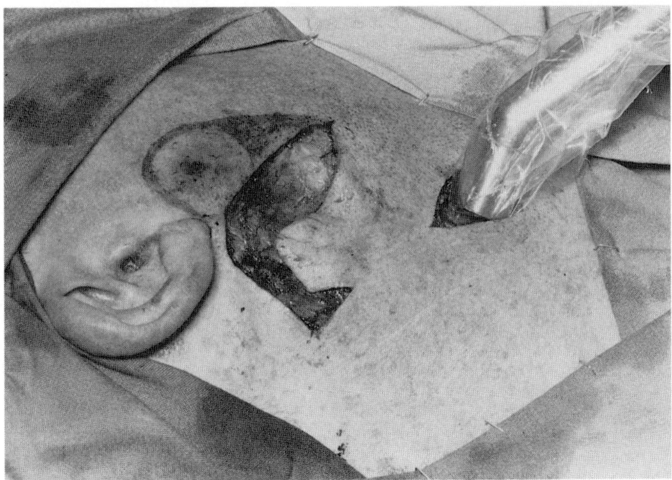

Figure 5.12 Using the gamma probe during surgery

The gamma probe helps to ensure that surgical dissection continues in the correct direction towards the 'hot' sentinel node. The probe is placed inside a sterile plastic sleeve and can thus be placed directly into the operative field. An incision has been made over the cross marking the site of one of the sentinel nodes in the neck in this patient (the same patient as in Figure 5.10) and the probe confirms the presence of a 'hot' sentinel node at this site. (An advancement flap to fill the defect created by wide excision of the primary melanoma site has already been elevated.)

body part to enhance lymphatic drainage. During surgery the sentinel node is then identified beneath the mark made on the skin at lymphoscintigraphy as the node receiving at least one blue channel and staining blue. The search for the sentinel node during surgery is facilitated by the *intraoperative use of the gamma probe*. The gamma probe helps to ensure that dissection continues toward the sentinel node, especially if the patient is obese when the sentinel node may be 10 cm deep to the skin mark. The sentinel node is identified during surgery as a blue staining node which is seen to have an afferent blue stained lymph channel and which is 'hot' with the gamma probe. The gamma probe is also useful to document a fall in residual node field counts to background levels after the sentinel node has been removed. We strongly contend that the use of all three techniques together is the most accurate method of ensuring that all sentinel nodes are visualised, located for surface marking and removed at surgery.

5.8 USING THE GAMMA DETECTING PROBE WITHOUT PREOPERATIVE LYMPHOSCINTIGRAPHY IN MELANOMA PATIENTS

Using a gamma detecting probe to find the 'hot' sentinel node in a draining node field after the injection of radiocolloid around the melanoma site without prior lymphoscintigraphy has certain attractions. There are cost savings if lymphoscintigraphy is omitted and the procedure can be performed in areas where high quality nuclear medicine services are not available. There are fewer appointments for the patient to coordinate and the timing of the injection of the radiocolloid is more in the surgeons control if he has a licence to handle radionuclides.

The disadvantages of using the gamma probe alone include, firstly, the risk that unusual lymphatic drainage patterns will be missed completely.[110] This would particularly involve many of the patients with trunk lesions especially on the back and around the nape of the neck, and would apply also for head and neck lesions. In these areas the lymphatic drainage patterns in individual patients can be quite complex with node fields overlying each other (Figure 5.13). Such complex lymphatic drainage can be accurately defined with high quality lymphoscintigraphy but would be extremely difficult if not impossible using a gamma detection probe without images.

A second problem for an approach which uses only a gamma probe is that node fields showing drainage only on the delayed scans might also be missed (see Figure 5.3). Thirdly not all radioactive nodes are sentinel nodes and many nodes particularly in the groin with lower limb injections rapidly receive tracer which has passed through the filter function of a sentinel node (see Figure 5.5).

These are not therefore sentinel nodes but can be quite radioactive even in the early dynamic phase. Removing all radioactive nodes in this situation will involve an unnecessarily extensive node dissection. As mentioned earlier, the visualisation of such second tier nodes is quite variable, occurring especially with melanoma sites on the foot, leg, thigh, hand and forearm. Using a count rate threshold on the probe in an attempt to distinguish sentinel nodes from second tier nodes has been advocated by some. However, sometimes a sentinel node has significantly less activity than second tier nodes in the same node field (see Figure 5.1), and thus this approach is not valid. It is also a disadvantage in some hospitals to have to inject the radioisotope in the surgical suite as this raises some radiation safety issues for the theatre staff which would not apply if the patient was injected in the nuclear medicine suite several hours or the day before surgery.

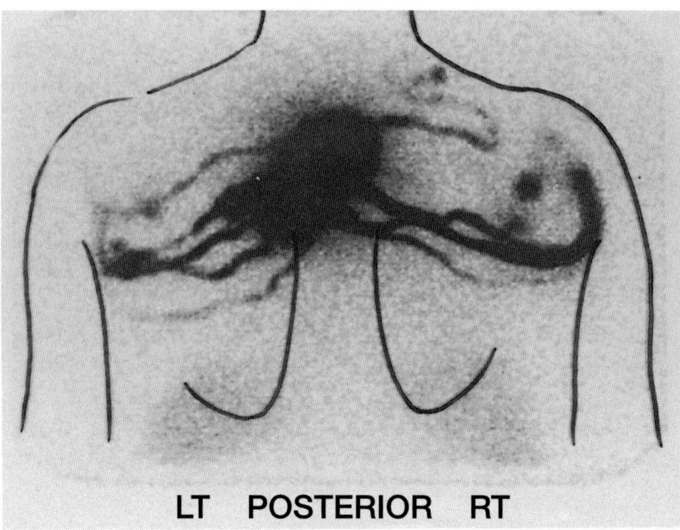

A

Figure 5.13 Complex drainage patterns need high resolution lymphoscintigraphy

On the dynamic image (A) multiple dominant channels are seen passing to the axilla and triangular intermuscular space bilaterally as well as over the shoulder to the right supraclavicular fossa.

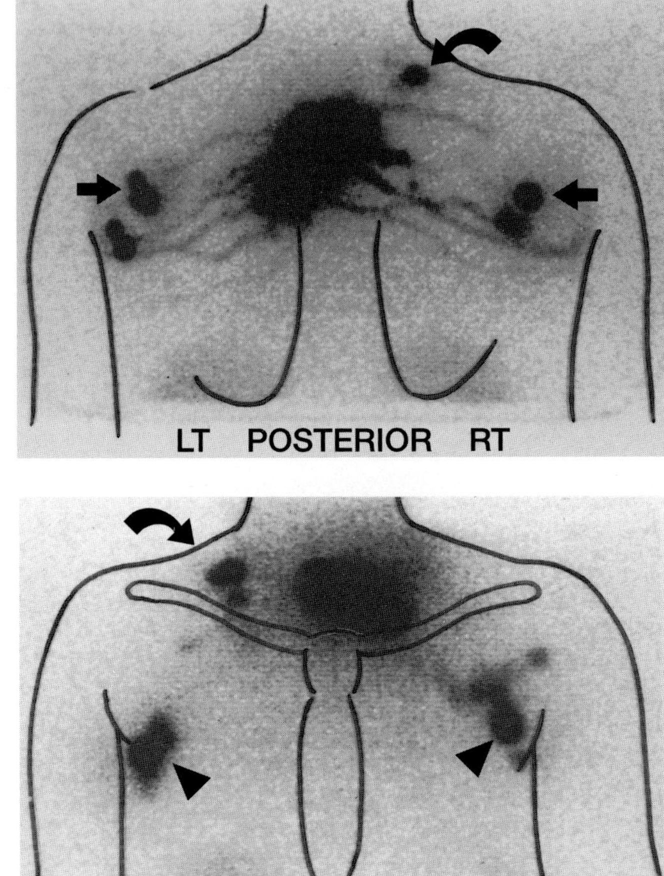

Figure 5.13 *Contined*

On the delayed scans (B and C) activity in sentinel nodes is seen in the triangular muscular space bilaterally (arrows), the axilla bilaterally (arrowheads) and the right supraclavicular fossa (curved arrow). The nodes in the axilla and triangular intermuscular space are close together and it would be extremely difficult to differentiate one from the other using a gamma probe alone without lymphoscintigraphy.

Chapter 6

PATTERNS OF LYMPHATIC DRAINAGE OF THE SKIN

6.1 TRUNK

Clinical prediction of the node fields which drain a particular part of the skin of the trunk is an uncertain process. Sappey[15] used mercury injected into the interstitial tissue and sometimes directly into the lymphatics of cadavers to define the zones of the trunk which he predicted would drain to the right and left axilla and the right and left groin nodes. These were defined by a demarcation line down the midline front and back and a transverse line around the waist from the umbilicus anteriorly to the second lumbar vertebra posteriorly (see Figure 2.3). Sappey suggested that these lines divided the trunk into 4 zones and that lymph drainage from the skin of the trunk would occur to the appropriate axilla or groin node field which lay within each zone and that drainage would not occur across these lines.

Earlier workers such as Mascagni[54] and some of Sappey's own disciples, Poirier, Cuneo and Delamere[32], suggested that drainage across the midline was possible, however this was ignored and Sappey's basic concepts were accepted as correct until the 1970s when others showed that there was a strip of skin along Sappey's lines about 5 cm wide within which drainage was uncertain.[11, 111] Drainage within this strip could be to either axilla or groin or to both. These authors still held that Sappey's predictions of lymphatic drainage would be accurate outside this narrow zone of uncertainty.

In 1953 Sherman and Ter-Pogossian[69] described a new technique called lymphoscintigraphy which allowed the lymphatic drainage patterns in individual patients to be accurately mapped. When this technique was applied to patients with melanoma and other malignancies on the skin of the trunk, it soon became clear that Sappey's lines did not define the draining node fields in many patients. Subsequent workers confirmed the extreme variability of lymphatic drainage from the skin of the trunk.[112–115] Norman et al.[116] defined and expanded new zones of ambiguity based on this increasing store of knowledge and

Eberbach[117] tried to combine data from several authors to further illustrate the extensive overlap of areas which drain to the various node fields.

In 1986 when we first began to perform lymphoscintigraphy in patients of the Sydney Melanoma Unit with cutaneous melanoma, we were using it to define the draining node field or fields in patients who had lesions in areas considered likely to have ambiguous drainage. These were mainly lesions on the trunk or the head and neck. Like others, we quickly observed the enormous variability in lymphatic drainage patterns from patient to patient from similar areas of the trunk and our potentially ambiguous zones on the trunk rapidly grew larger and larger until we came to regard almost any lesion on the trunk as having potentially ambiguous drainage (see Figures 4.3, 4.4 and 4.5). Then in 1992 Morton et al.[104] described a method of locating the sentinel lymph node in patients with melanoma using injections of blue dye. From this time we began using lymphoscintigraphy to locate the sentinel nodes in each draining node field as well as defining the drainage pattern in each patient. This meant that the technique was relevant for all patients and we began to perform lymphoscintigraphy in patients who had what was thought previously to be unambiguous drainage, such as from the upper and lower limbs. As a result we now have data on the lymphatic drainage of the skin for almost 2000 patients with lesion sites all over the skin.

Our data show that drainage in the directions indicated by Sappey's lines is more likely to be correct for lesions on the anterior trunk than for those on the posterior trunk (see Figure 4.3). It can be seen that drainage across the midline is not common from the anterior trunk but is frequent from the posterior trunk and often from a site well away from the midline. Drainage across Sappey's horizontal line around the waist from sites on the low back to the axilla is also not uncommon, and drainage from above Sappey's line to groin nodes can also occur (Figure 6.1). Drainage from the skin of the trunk usually includes the axilla but exceptions occur (see Figure 4.6).

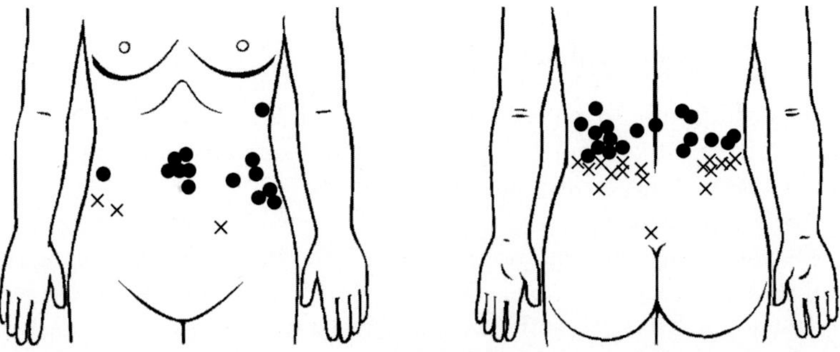

Figure 6.1 Sites draining across Sappey's horizontal line around the waist Dots show sites draining to the groin across Sappey's line. Crosses show sites draining up to the axilla across Sappey's line.

We have found unusual patterns of lymphatic drainage from the trunk of some patients. In 20% of patients, for example, lymphatics drain from the peri-umbilical area to a right costal margin interval node before passing towards the midline and then through the chest wall to right internal mammary nodes[99] (Figure 6.2). We recently saw a patient who showed drainage to a similar left costal margin sentinel node from the skin above the umbilicus and to the left of midline (Figure 6.3).

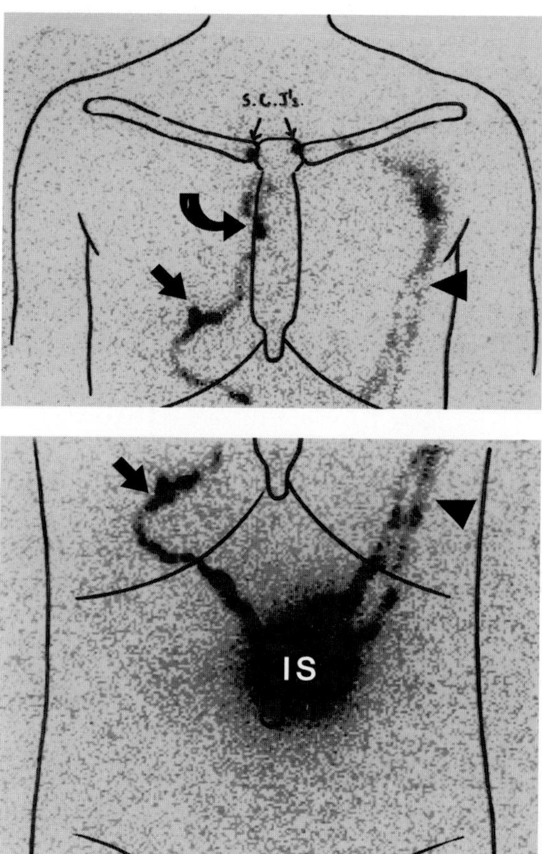

Figure 6.2 Drainage from the periumbilical area to a costal margin node and on to internal mammary nodes

Dynamic scans show two dominant channels passing from the injection site (IS) towards the left axilla (arrowhead) and a single channel coursing over the right costal margin to a subcutaneous sentinel node (arrow). The channel then passes through the chest wall to the right internal mammary chain (curved arrow).

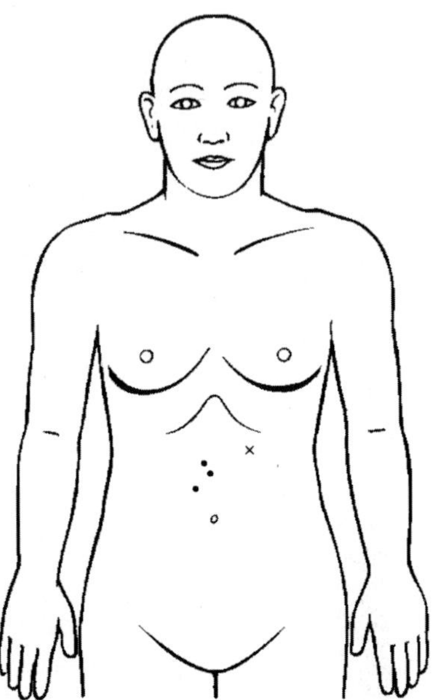

Figure 6.3 Sites draining to the right and left costal margin sentinel node then onwards to the internal mammary chain

Dots show sites draining to the right costal margin node and the cross shows the primary site which drained to a left costal margin node. These are all clustered around an area just above the umbilicus.

In 26% of patients lymphatics drain from the skin of the back to nodes in the triangular inter-muscular space node field[96] (Figure 6.4). This drainage can be unilateral or bilateral (Figure 6.5). Drainage to this node field is perhaps the most important unusual pathway to look for when performing lymphoscintigraphy to locate sentinel nodes. If drainage to this node field is overlooked then sentinel nodes will be missed in one in four patients with melanomas on the back.

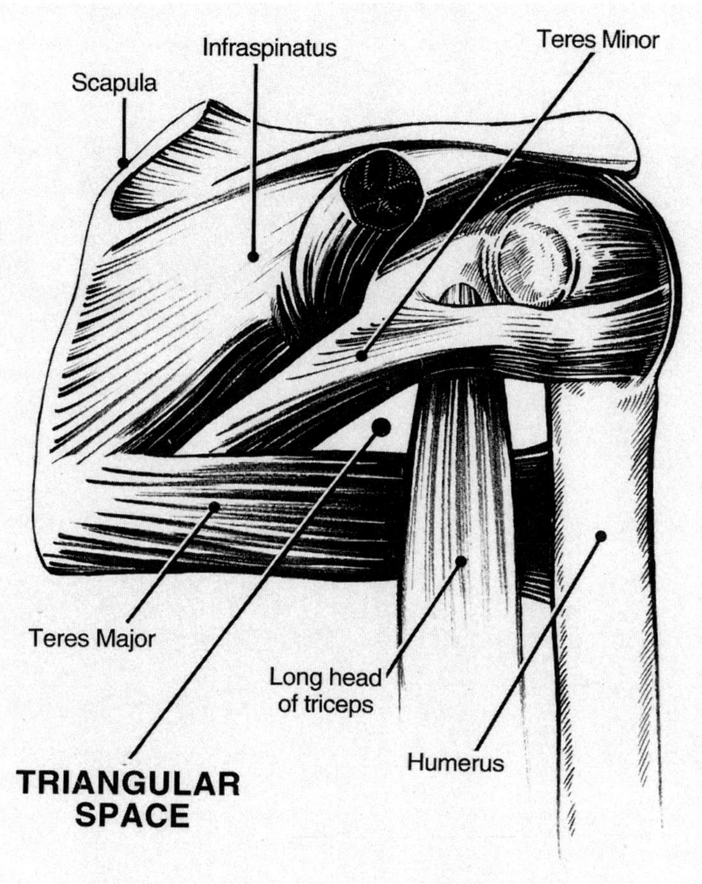

A

Figure 6.4 Bilateral drainage to the triangular intermuscular space

A: Schematic diagram of the right triangular intermuscular space. B: Dynamic image showing dominant channels passing from the injection site (IS) on the upper back just to the right of midline to the triangular intermuscular space bilaterally (arrows) and to the right axilla (arrowhead). C: Delayed posterior scan showing sentinel nodes in the TIS bilaterally (arrows). Notice how faint these are on the anterior image (D) due to attenuation through the patients body. A faint right axillary sentinel node was also present best seen in the lateral view (not shown).

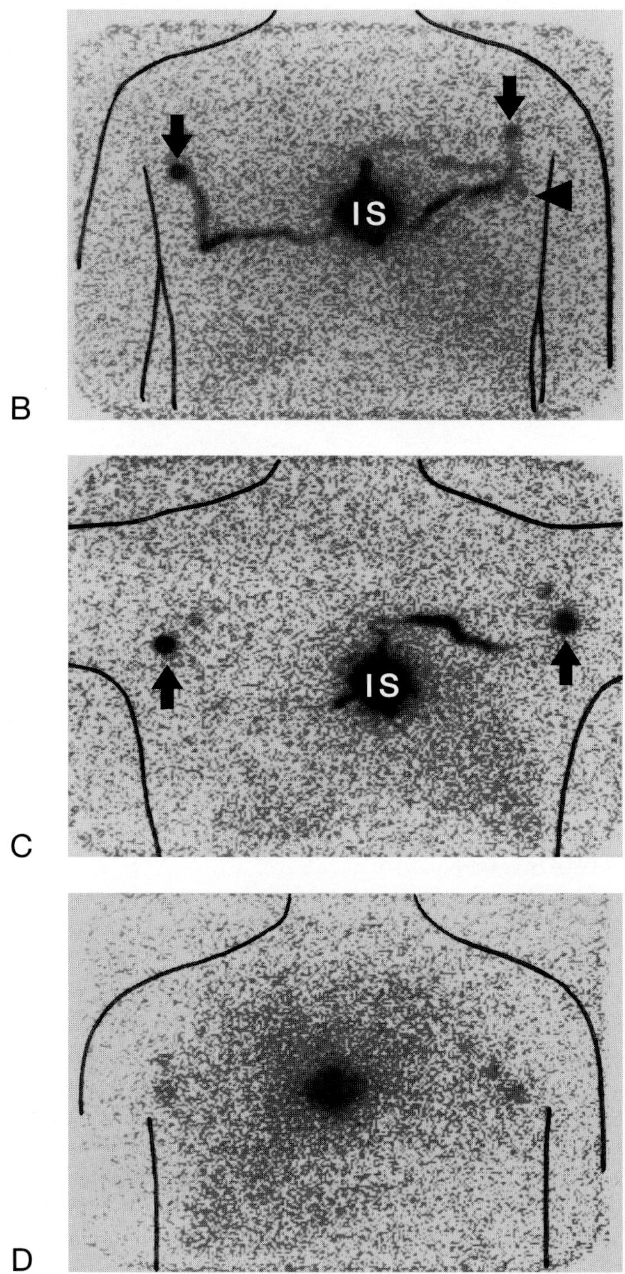

Figure 6.4 *Continued*

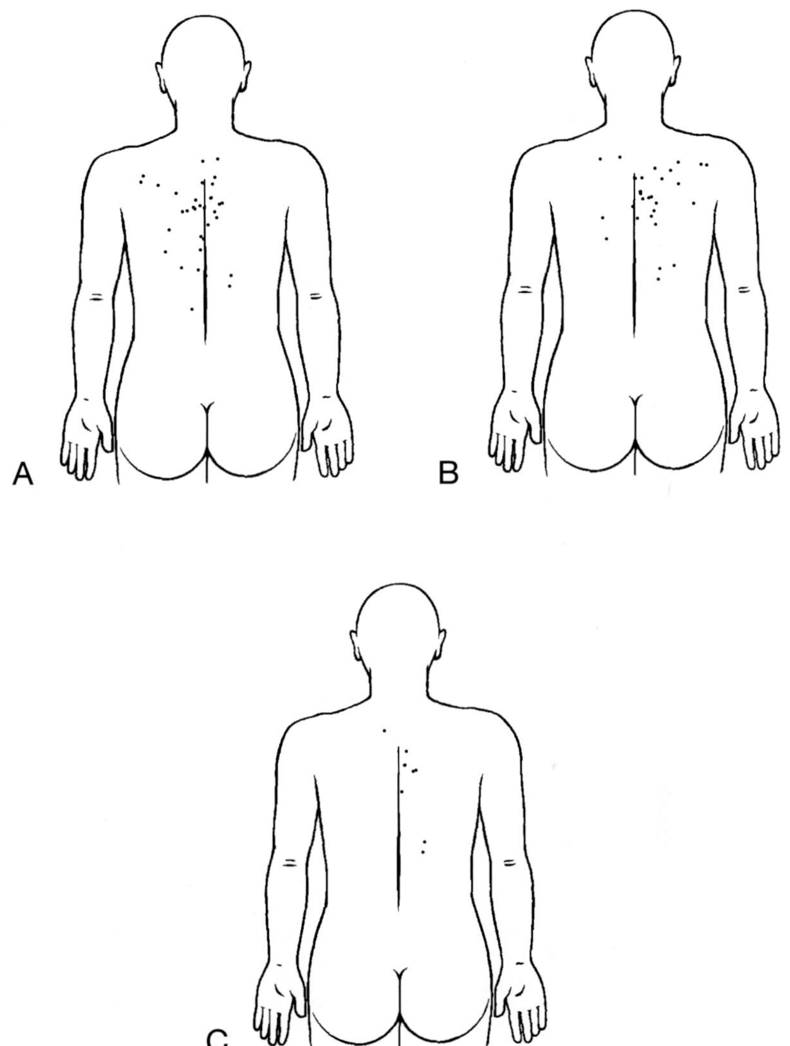

Figure 6.5 Skin sites which drain to the triangular intermuscular space
Sites which drain to the left TIS (A), the right TIS (B) and both right and left TIS (C).

Some patients have lymphatic channels which pass from the skin of the posterior loin superiorly towards the midline and then through the body wall to paravertebral lymph nodes and then upwards towards the thoracic duct (Figure 6.6). We have also seen a lymph channel pass directly through the body wall in the posterior loin to nodes in the retroperitoneal space, with onward drainage from there to paravertebral nodes[98] (Figure 6.7). Most of these patients also have some drainage to the usual node fields of the axilla and groin but we have encountered three patients who had drainage only to paravertebral nodes, with no drainage at all to the axilla or groin[118]. The primary melanoma sites which showed drainage to paravertebral and retroperitoneal nodes are displayed in Figure 6.8.

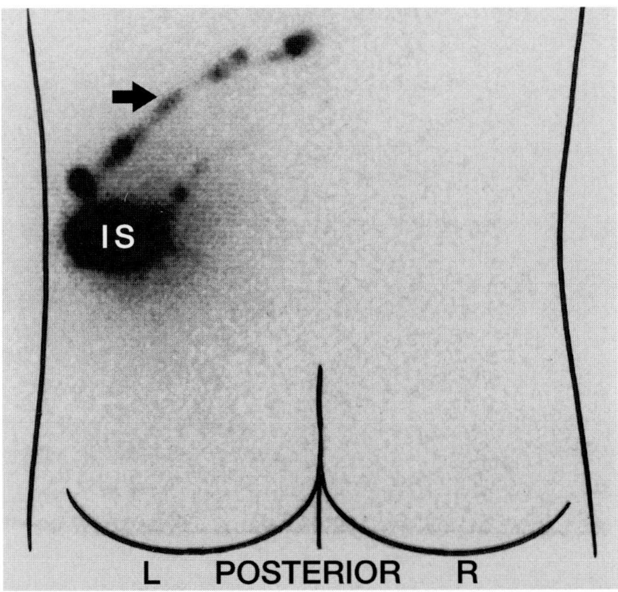

Figure 6.6 Direct Drainage to Paravertebral Nodes

On the dynamic image (A) a channel can be seen passing from the injection site (IS) up towards the midline (arrow). On the delayed scans (B and C) tracer is seen in paravertebral nodes (arrow) and in left groin nodes (arrowhead). Faint tracer is also seen high in the thorax in the region of the thoracic duct (curved arrow). This thoracic duct activity is almost always seen in patients who show direct drainage to paravertebral nodes and its presence should alert the physician to the possibility of such a drainage pattern. The imaging protocol should then be altered to include a search for activity in paravertebral lymph nodes.

B

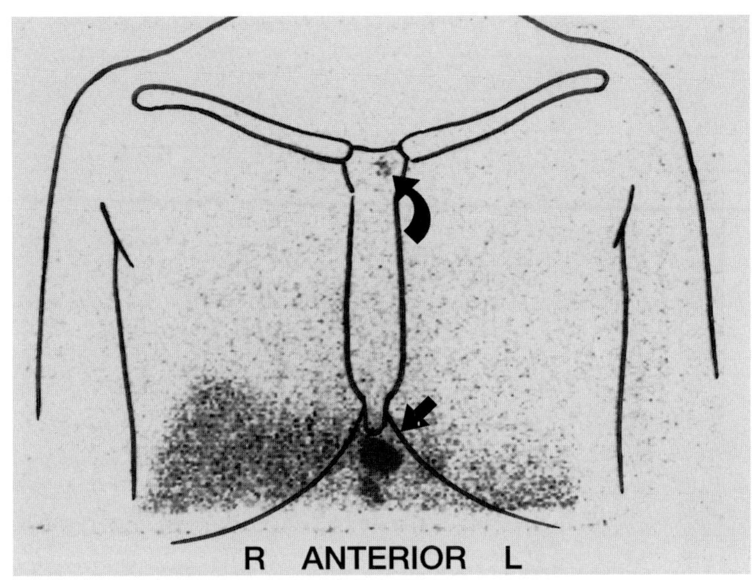

C

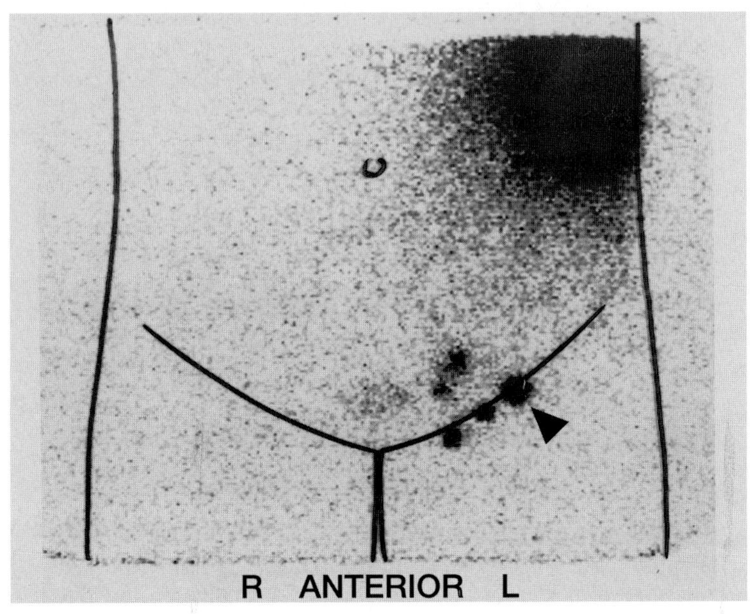

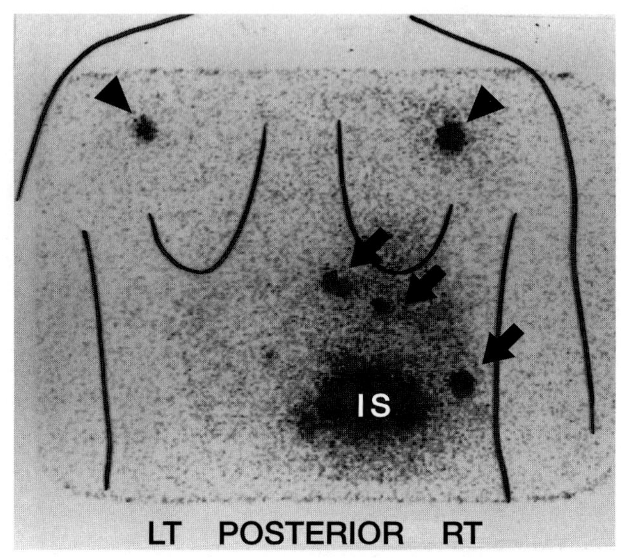

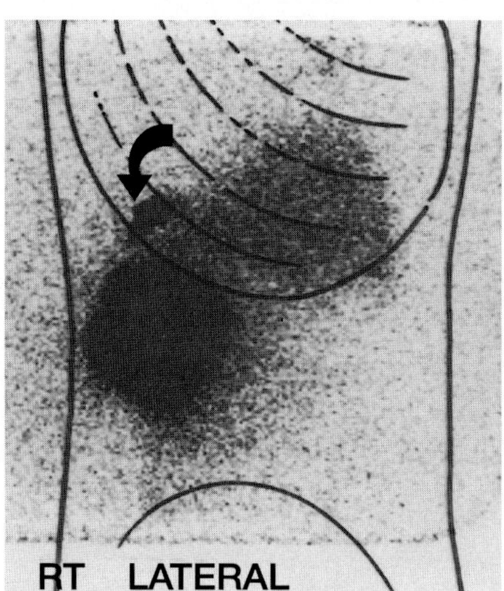

Figure 6.7 Direct drainage to retroperitoneal nodes

This patient with an injection site on the mid back to the right of midline shows in (A) drainage directly to sentinel nodes in the axilla bilaterally (arrowheads) and retroperitoneal nodes (arrows). In the lateral view (B) the depth of the node from the skin of the posterior body wall can be seen. This node (curved arrow) lay 8 cm deep to the skin of the back.

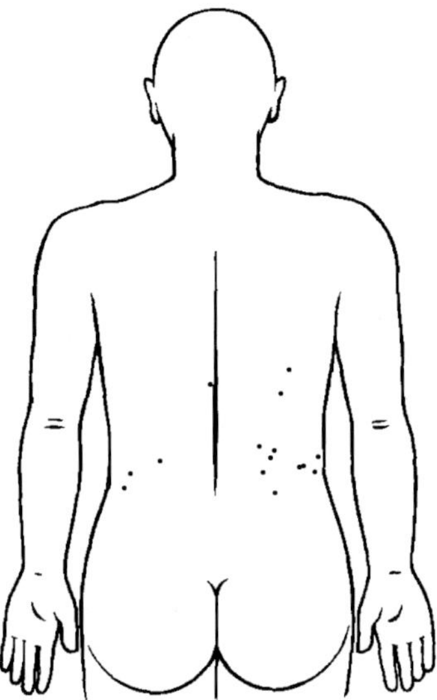

Figure 6.8 Sites draining to paravertebral and retroperitoneal nodes
Drainage to paravertebral and retroperitoneal nodes occurs mainly from sites on the posterior loin, with the occasional site higher in the midline and on the posterior chest showing this pattern.

Interval nodes in the subcutaneous tissue of the trunk are most common low in the mid-axillary line (see Figure 5.2), along channels passing towards the axilla. They are also found along the back, as channels pass up and towards the midline before passing through the body wall to paravertebral nodes. Interval nodes are also often seen along the path of channels passing up towards posterior triangle (Level V cervical) nodes from sites on the upper back, and on the posterior buttocks in the line of channels heading towards groin nodes from sites on the low back (Figure 6.9).

We have performed lymphatic mapping on 731 patients with primary sites on the trunk, 610 of them on the posterior trunk and 121 on the anterior trunk. The results of our findings for posterior trunk primary sites are summarised in Table 6.1.

Of those who showed drainage to the axilla in this group of patients with posterior trunk primary sites, there were 186 patients who showed bilateral axillary drainage (Figure 6.10). Of those who showed drainage to groin nodes there were 16 who had bilateral groin node drainage (see Figure 4.4). The incidence of drainage from the posterior trunk to the triangular intermuscular space

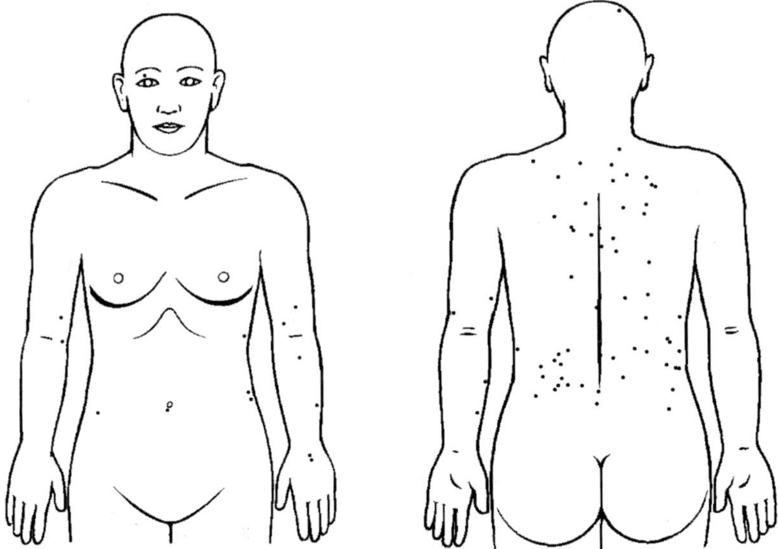

Figure 6.9 Sites on the anterior and posterior torso which have drainage to interval nodes

Drainage to interval nodes can occur from sites over much of the back as well as occasional sites on the head and arms.

Table 6.1 Posterior trunk primary sites

Draining node field	*Number of patients*	*% of total*
Axilla	554	91
Groin	63	10
Supraclavicular	84	14
Triangular intermuscular space	55	9
Paravertebral	15	2.5
Cervical Level III	1	<1
Cervical Level IV	8	1
Cervical Level V	40	7
Occipital	1	<1
Interval nodes	56	9

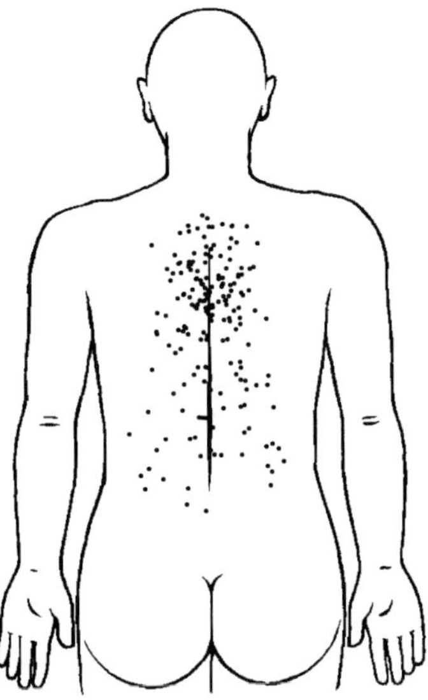

Figure 6.10 Sites on the posterior trunk which drain to both axillae

lymph nodes is only about 9% when our whole data set is analysed, however, our earlier studies were performed using an imaging protocol which did not look for sentinel nodes in this node field. It was after we first observed drainage to this node field several years ago that we altered out protocol so that this node field was always checked for sentinel nodes in patients with back lesions. We now detect nodes in this field in approximately 20% of such patients. In the 15 patients who showed drainage through the posterior abdominal wall directly to paravertebral nodes there were 3 who also showed drainage to retroperitoneal nodes. Eight of the patients with drainage to the triangular intermuscular space showed drainage to these nodes bilaterally and 10 patients showed drainage to the supraclavicular nodes bilaterally. Five of the 40 patients with drainage to posterior triangle nodes (Cervical Level V) had bilateral drainage to these nodes.

The results in our patients with anterior trunk primary melanoma sites are summarised in Table 6.2.

In patients with anterior trunk primary sites who showed drainage to the axilla, 21 had bilateral drainage (Figure 6.11) while only one patient had bilateral drainage to the supraclavicular fossae. A noticeable difference between the anterior and posterior trunk drainage is the significantly smaller percentage of patients with anterior trunk primary sites who show drainage to the supraclavicular fossa, 6% for the anterior trunk versus 14% for the posterior trunk.

Table 6.2 Anterior trunk primary sites

Draining node field	*Number of patients*	*% of total*
Axilla	98	81
Groin	22	18
Supraclavicular	7	6
Triangular intermuscular space	0	0
Paravertebral	0	0
Cervical Level II	1	<1
Cervical Level III	3	2.5
Cervical Level IV	1	<1
Cervical Level V	0	0
Occipital	0	0
Costal margin	5	4
Interval nodes	6	5

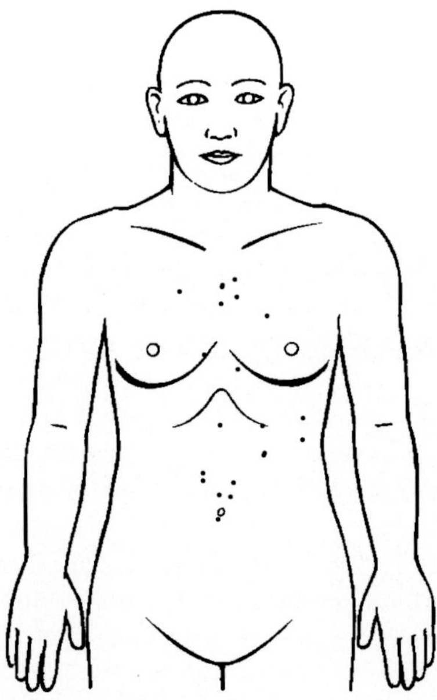

Figure 6.11 Sites on the anterior trunk which drain to both axillae

We did not expect to see drainage from the anterior trunk to the triangular intermuscular space and this was not found. No drainage was seen to Level V cervical nodes or occipital nodes and it appears that direct drainage to paravertebral nodes does not occur from the anterior trunk. We did not see any patient show drainage from the skin of the anterior trunk directly to intramammary nodes, though this did occur via right and left costal margin nodes in 4% of patients. Interval nodes were seen less often on the anterior trunk compared to the posterior trunk.

6.1.1 BASE OF NECK

The skin around the base of the neck is an area which has particularly unpredictable drainage patterns. Drainage can occur to supraclavicular nodes (Figure 4.5), occipital nodes, cervical nodes (Level II, III, IV and V), (Figure 6.12 and Figure 6.13) triangular intermuscular space nodes (see Figure 6.5) and axillary nodes. It is not uncommon for lymph channels to pass over the shoulder from the back to supraclavicular nodes (Figure 6.14). The drainage pattern from the base of the neck area usually involves multiple draining node fields.

We have now studied 154 patients with primary melanoma sites in this area. Our findings are summarised in Table 6.3.

In 24 patients drainage was to both axillae (see Figure 6.10 and 6.11), while 11 had bilateral drainage to the supraclavicular fossae (see Figure 4.5), 3 bilateral drainage to Level V cervical nodes, 1 bilateral drainage to Level IV cervical nodes and 1 bilateral drainage to triangular intermuscular space sentinel nodes. Drainage from the posterior base of neck to both supraclavicular fossae occurred from only a very small area of the skin of the upper back around the midline (see Figure 4.5). In 124 patients the primary site was on the posterior aspect of the base of the neck and 53 of them (43%) showed drainage over the shoulders to sentinel nodes in the supraclavicular fossa. Seven of these patients (6%) had drainage over the shoulders to cervical nodes at Level III or IV. There was drainage across the midline in 40 patients (32%) to sentinel nodes in a total of 53 node fields.

In the 30 patients who had primary sites on the base of the neck anteriorly there were 6 (20%) who showed drainage across the midline. Five (17%) showed drainage up the neck to cervical Level II or III nodes (Figure 6.15) and 25 (83%) showed drainage down to the axilla. Axillary drainage was bilateral in 3 patients while 1 patient had bilateral drainage to supraclavicular nodes and 1 had bilateral drainage to cervical Level III nodes.

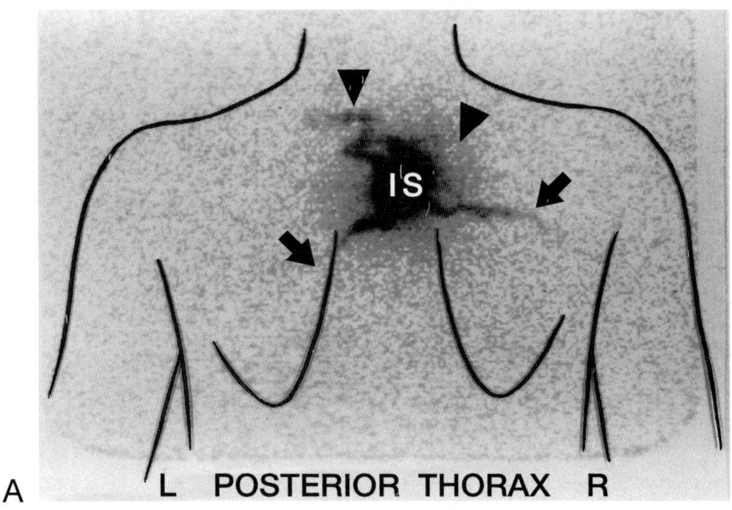

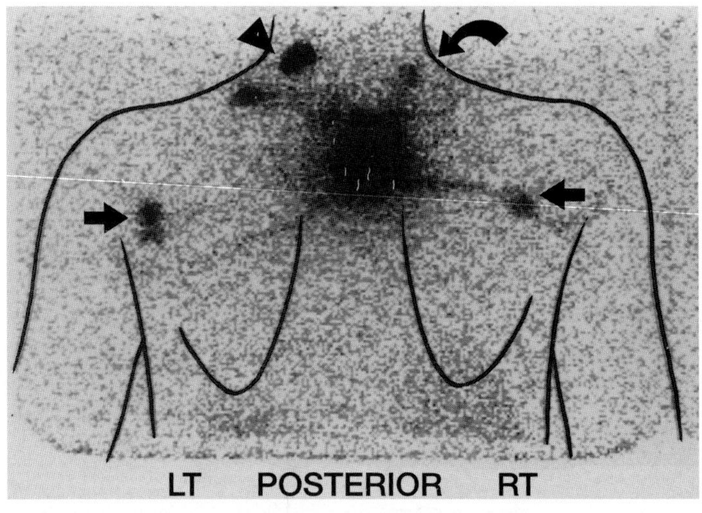

Figure 6.12 Drainage from the back to posterior triangle nodes

The injection site (IS) is seen on the dynamic scan (A) and channels are seen passing towards each axilla (arrows). Early channels are also seen passing superiorly (arrowheads). On the delayed scan (B) sentinel nodes are seen in the axilla bilaterally (arrows) and there is a sentinel node in a left posterior triangle Level V node (arrowhead). A sentinel node was also present in the right supraclavicular fossa. This is only faintly seen on the posterior view (curved arrow).

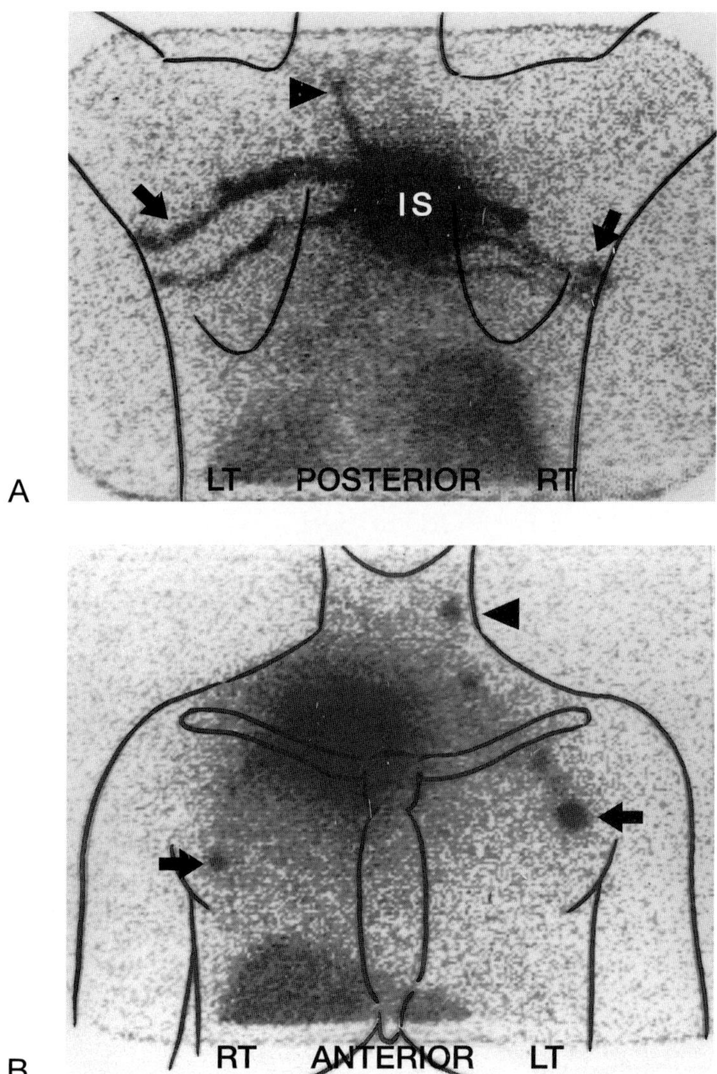

Figure 6.13 Drainage from back to Level III cervical nodes across the midline

The injection site (IS) is seen on the dynamic image (A). Three dominant channels on each side converge to a single sentinel node in each axilla (arrows) and a single dominant channel crosses the midline on its way up to the mid left neck (arrowhead). On the delayed scan (B) there is a single sentinel node in each axilla (arrows) and a sentinel node on the left at cervical Level III (arrowhead).

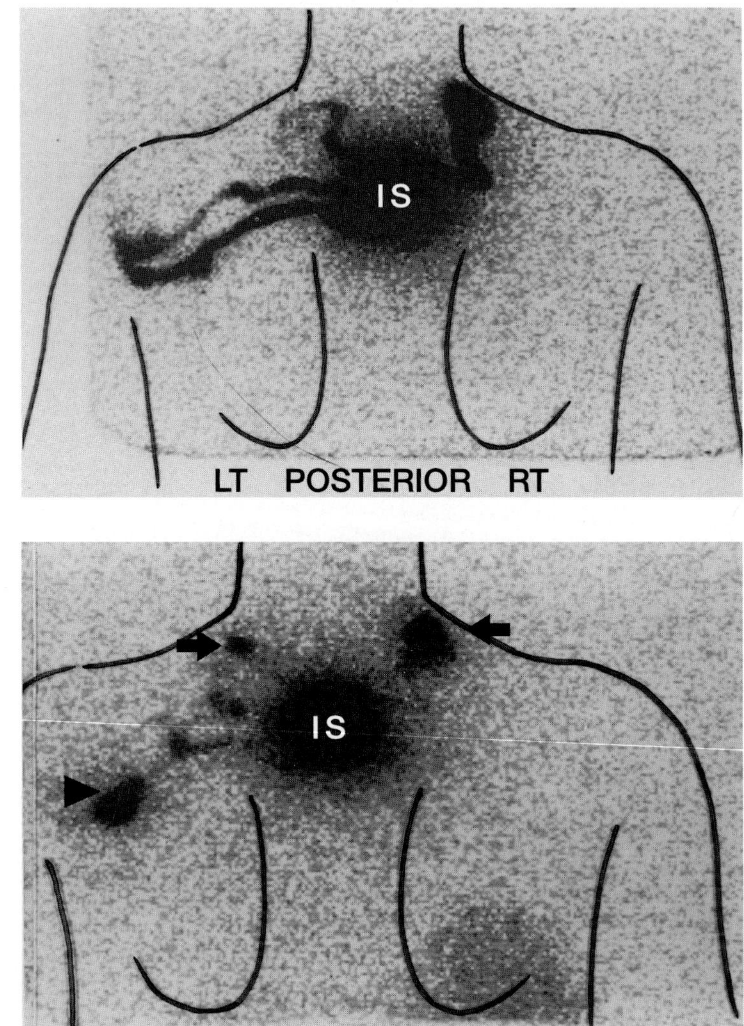

Figure 6.14 Drainage from the back to right and left supraclavicular nodes

The dynamic scan (A) shows 2 dominant channels passing towards the left axilla from the injection site (IS). Channels are also seen passing over the shoulders to the supraclavicular fossae bilaterally. The delayed scans (B and C) show sentinel nodes in the supraclavicular fossae bilaterally (arrows) and 2 sentinel nodes in the left axilla (arrowheads).

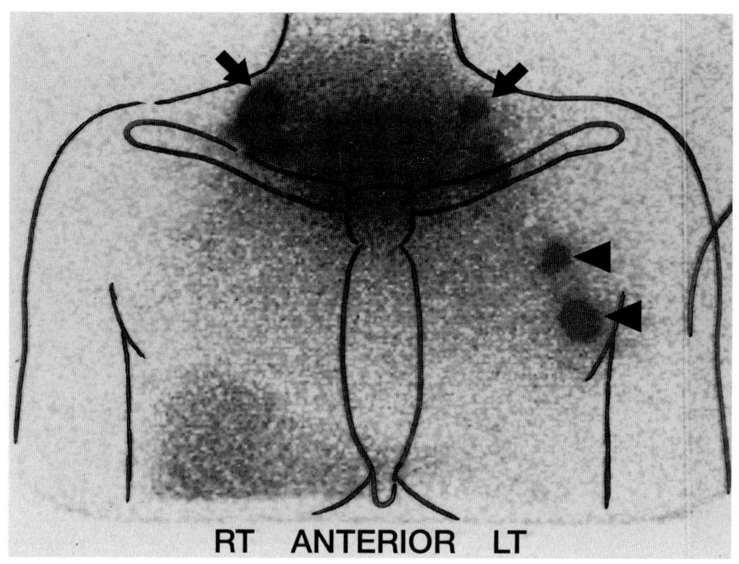

Figure 6.14 *Continued*

Table 6.3 Base of neck primary sites

Draining node field	*Number of patients*	*% of total*
Axilla	134	87
Supraclavicular	68	44
Triangular intermuscular space	11	7
Cervical Level II	2	1
Cervical Level III	4	3
Cervical Level IV	8	5
Cervical Level V	27	18
Occipital	1	0.5
Interval nodes	9	6

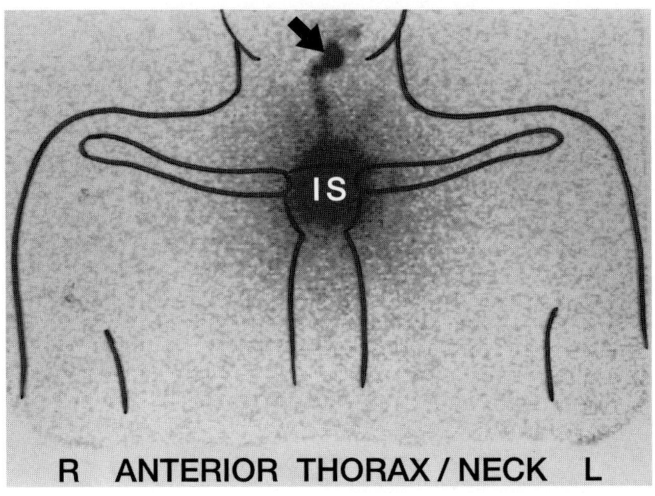

A

B

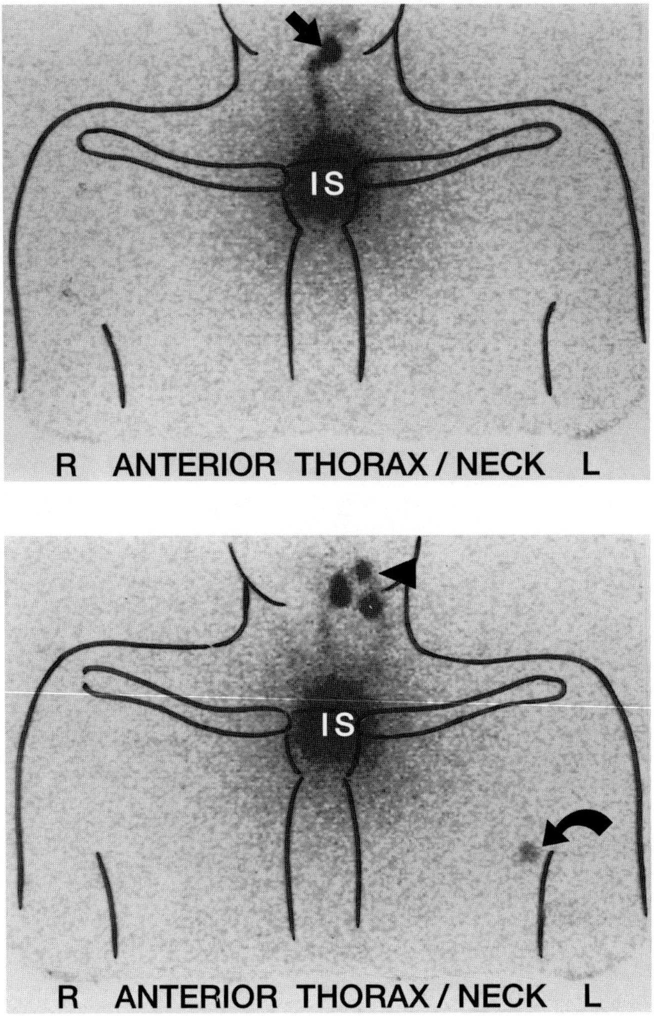

Figure 6.15 Drainage from the anterior base of neck to Level II and Level III cervical nodes

A: The injection site (IS) over the manubrium is seen. On the dynamic image a channel passes up the neck to a Level III node (arrow) and on the delayed scan (B) a separate channel is seen passing to a Level II node (arrowhead). Drainage also occurs to a left axillary node (curved arrow).

6.2 HEAD AND NECK

In the past, guidelines have been proposed for clinical prediction of lymphatic drainage patterns from the skin of the head and neck.[119, 120] These have suggested that drainage from the face is to ipsilateral parotid and Level I–III cervical nodes, from the anterior scalp to parotid and Level I–III nodes, from the posterior scalp to occipital and Level II–V nodes and from the coronal midline scalp to parotid and Level I–V nodes. Drainage from the skin of the anterior upper neck would be expected to be to parotid and Level I–IV nodes, while the anterior lower neck would be expected to drain to Level III–V nodes. Drainage from the skin of the posterior upper neck would be expected to be to occipital and Level II–V nodes, while drainage from the posterior lower neck is predicted to be to Levels III–V nodes. The coronal upper neck would include parotid and Level I–V nodes, while the ear would be expected to drain to the parotid and Level I–V nodes.

However, when we used lymphoscintigraphy to examine lymphatic flow patterns in the head and neck[102], we found that lymphatic drainage was discordant with clinical prediction in 33 of 97 (34%) patients studied. A total of 21 patients (22%) had drainage to nodes other than the parotid and the 5 standard neck levels. In 13 this was to postauricular nodes and in 5 this was to occipital nodes. The postauricular nodes are not usually resected in an elective radical node dissection for malignant disease of the head and neck and the occipital nodes are only resected when the primary site is on the posterior scalp or upper neck. We found drainage from the face and anterior scalp to postauricular nodes in 3 of 35 patients. Other areas which drained to postauricular nodes were the ear (3 of 11 patients) and posterior scalp (4 of 18 patients). We also found drainage from the posterior scalp to parotid nodes (2 of 18 patients), drainage from the anterior scalp direct to Level IV nodes (2 of 19 patients) and from the face to Level IV and V nodes (2 of 31 patients). We observed drainage from the base of the neck to parotid, Level II cervical and occipital nodes. Contralateral drainage across the midline was seen in 5 of 31 patients with face lesions, and in 1 of 8 patients with lesions on the upper neck. Five patients had drainage from the posterior lower neck to the axilla and one patient had drainage from the left anterior neck base to the left axilla (Figure 6.16).

We have now mapped the patterns of lymphatic drainage in 205 patients who had primary melanoma sites on the head and neck. The node fields which received drainage from these sites are summarised in Table 6.4.

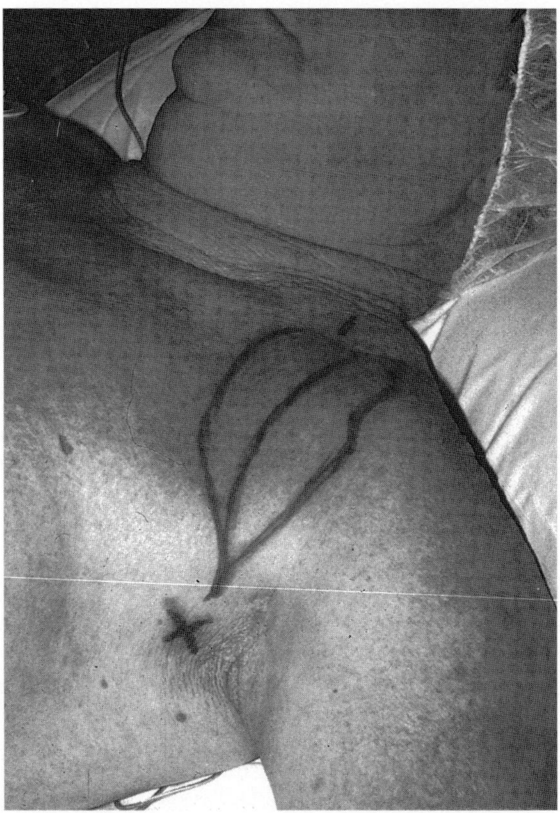

Figure 6.16 Drainage from the base of the neck to the axilla

A patient with a primary site on the anterior neck base which drained to the axilla. Several channels converged towards a single sentinel node in the left axilla.

Table 6.4 Head and neck primary sites

Draining node field	*Number of patients*	*% of total*
Preauricular (parotid)	79	39
Postauricular	27	13
Occipital	22	11
Cervical Level I	32	16
Cervical Level II	127	62
Cervical Level III	28	14
Cervical Level IV	35	17
Cervical Level V	38	19
Submental	4	2
Supraclavicular	28	14
Axilla	6	3
Triangular intermuscular space	1	0.5
Interval nodes	7	3.5
No drainage	1	0.5

Drainage occurred across the midline in 30 patients (15%) (Figure 6.17) and the coronal line across the head defined by the position of the ears was crossed in 27 patients (13%). (Figure 6.18 and 6.19) Direct drainage down the neck to sentinel nodes beyond those normally expected occurred in 42 patients (21%). (Figure 6.20) Unexpected drainage also occurred from primary sites low in the neck up to sentinel nodes in the occipital, preauricular, postauricular, Level I cervical or Level II cervical nodes in 28 patients (14%) (Figure 6.21).

It is thus clear that any attempt to make clinical predictions about lymphatic drainage pathways in patients with head and neck melanomas is unrealistic. If these predictions are used to determine the site and extent of lymph node surgery the surgeon will fail to remove nodes potentially containing metastatic disease in 1 in 3 patients. As with many other body sites, it appears that rational surgical management of draining lymph nodes in patients with malignant disease that spreads via the lymphatics is not possible unless preoperative lymphatic mapping using lymphoscintigraphy is performed.

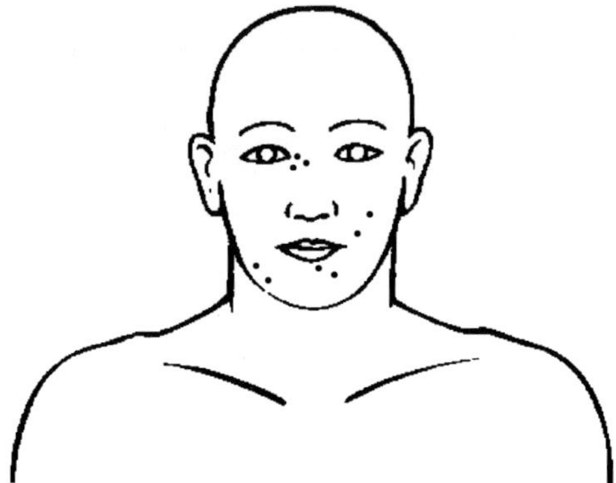

Figure 6.17 Sites which drain across the midline of the face to contralateral nodes

Dots show melanoma sites which had contralateral drainage. Such contralateral drainage is possible from the peri-oral area, the cheek and around the nose and eye.

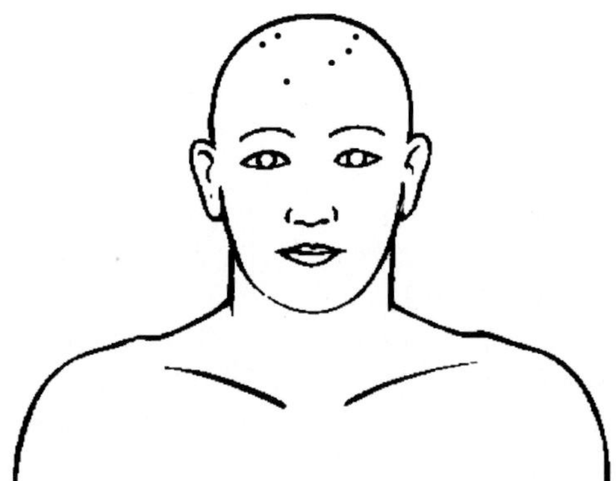

Figure 6.18 Sites which drain from the anterior scalp to postauricular nodes

Dots show melanoma sites which drained to postauricular nodes. Drainage to the postauricular nodes can occur from any part of the anterior scalp. These nodes are not removed in standard neck dissections for face or anterior scalp melanomas.

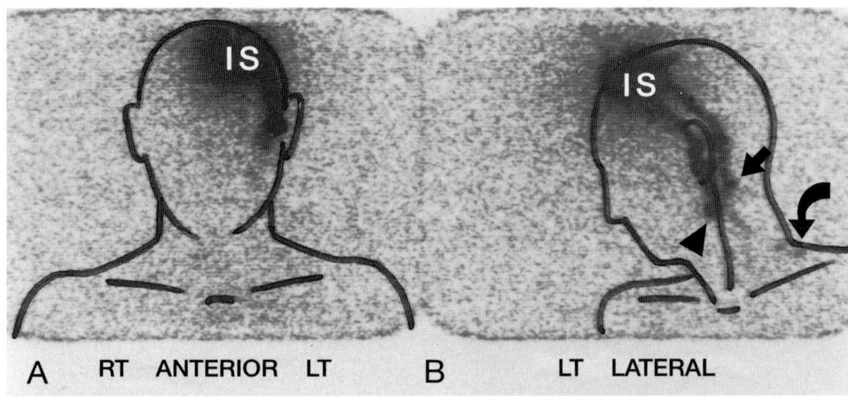

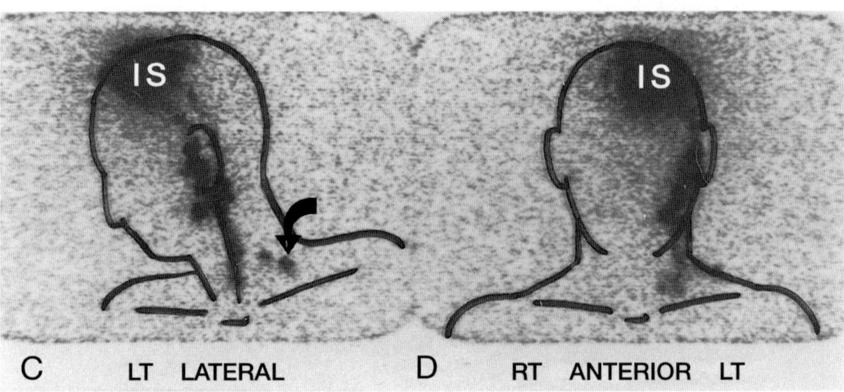

Figure 6.19 Anterior scalp melanoma site draining to postauricular nodes

The injection site (IS) around the melanoma is seen on the left anterior scalp. On dynamic imaging (A) 2 dominant channels are seen, 1 passing in front of the left ear to a parotid node (arrowhead) and 1 passing behind the ear to a postauricular node (arrow). These are both sentinel nodes. The postauricular nodes are not normally resected in melanoma surgery of the head and neck. In this patient second tier nodes are seen in the left supraclavicular fossa (curved arrow on B).

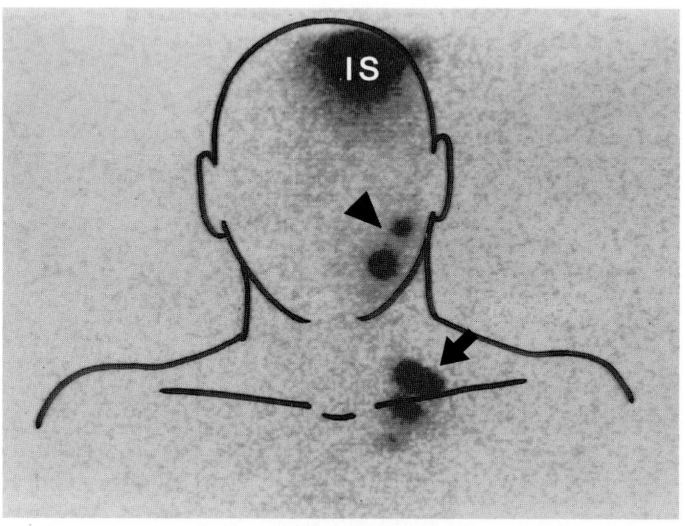

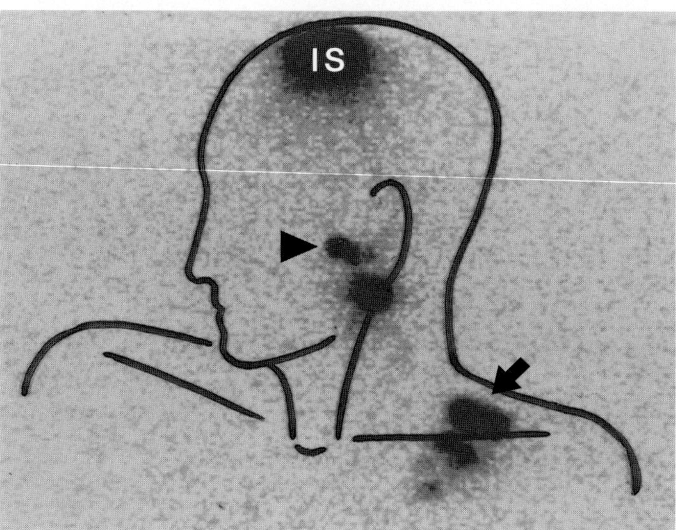

Figure 6.20 Direct drainage from the scalp to sentinel nodes in the supraclavicular fossa

The injection site (IS) on the left anterior scalp is seen. On dynamic imaging there were dominant channels which passed directly to left supraclavicular nodes (arrow) and separate channels which passed to left parotid nodes (arrowhead). The supraclavicular nodes are thus sentinel nodes in this patient.

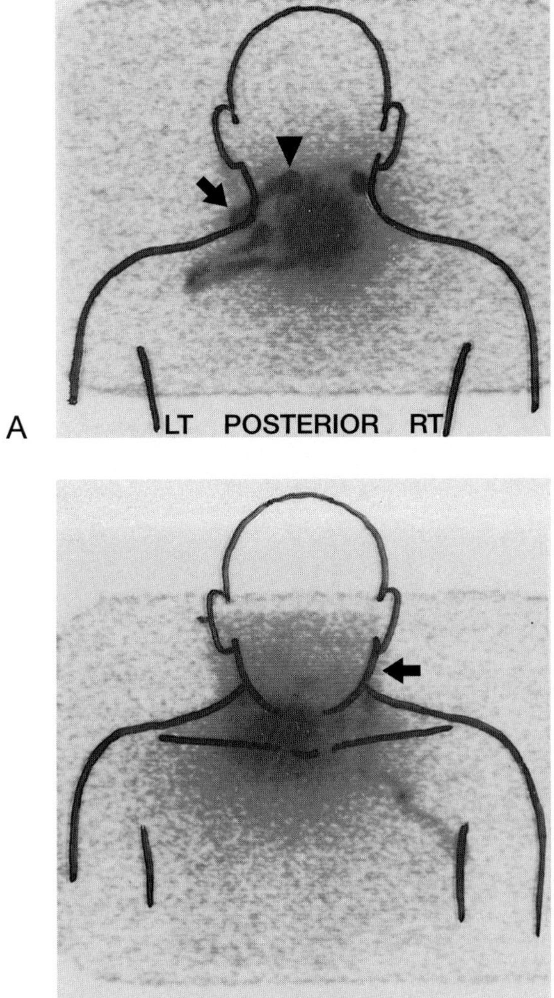

Figure 6.21 Drainage from the base of the neck posteriorly to Level II cervical nodes

This patient with a lesion on the base of the neck posteriorly showed a complex drainage pattern (A and B) which included drainage upwards to a left cervical Level II node (arrow). Drainage also occurred to the left axilla, right and left neck nodes, and upwards in the posterior neck to a low occipital node (arrowhead).

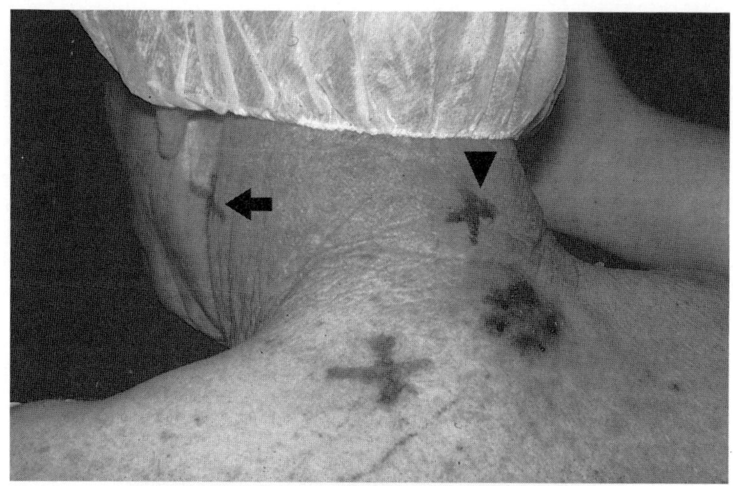

C

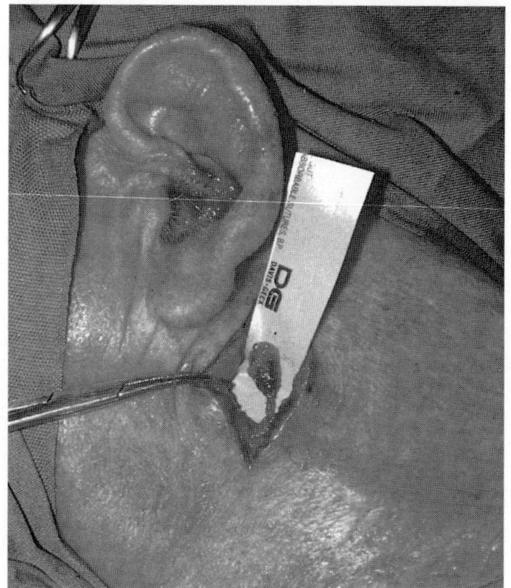

D

Figure 6.21 *Continued*

All of the sentinel nodes were found and stained blue (D), however the only node positive for metastasis was the occipital node above the injection sites posteriorly (arrowhead on C).

6.3 UPPER LIMB

Standard accounts of the anatomy of upper limb lymphatic vessels have been largely based on work by Rouviere[121]. Superficial and deep systems were described and the superficial system was divided into lateral and medial groups of lymph vessels. The lateral group was said to pass up the lateral aspect of the forearm with the cephalic vein while the medial group passed medially with the basilic vein. These medial channels were said to sometimes pass to epitrochlear nodes above the elbow, though the majority passed superiorly to the lateral axillary nodes. Many of the lateral group were said to pass medially at the elbow to continue on with the medial group, while those channels which persisted in a lateral course stayed with the cephalic vein and eventually reached the deltopectoral nodes. Efferent channels were then said to pass on to the subclavicular (apical) axillary nodes or the inferior cervical nodes. A complex system of drainage was described with channels passing from one group of axillary nodes to the next with most passing finally to the apical nodes before passing on to form the subclavian trunk, which itself drains directly into the jugular trunk, the junction of the internal jugular and subclavian vein or the thoracic duct.[68]

The pattern of lymph drainage suggested above is not the situation we have observed from the skin of the upper limb, based on lymphoscintigraphy studies. Most skin sites on the upper limb drain to the axilla and we have never seen direct drainage to deltopectoral nodes. As in other parts of the body we have found lymph drainage from the upper limb to be extremely variable, with channels passing directly to sentinel nodes in many parts of the axilla. There is most commonly only one sentinel node in the axilla (average 1.3 sentinel nodes[103]) with upper limb injections.

From the arm some patients have direct drainage to supraclavicular nodes and rarely to cervical nodes. Drainage from the forearm is usually exclusively to the axilla though we have seen 4 patients with additional direct drainage to supraclavicular nodes[100] from the proximal forearm, and one with drainage from the dorsum of the wrist directly to a supraclavicular node (Figure 6.22).

Drainage to epitrochlear nodes[122] occurs less often than had previously been thought, however it is important to perform a full delayed acquisition over the epitrochlear region during lymphoscintigraphy to ensure that any sentinel nodes in this field are detected (Figure 4.8). Our original protocol called for a full acquisition only if tracer was seen on the persistance scope. Using this approach in 109 patients with lesion sites on the forearm or hand, only 4 showed drainage to an epitrochlear node, an incidence of approximately 4%. Over the last 15 months we have changed our imaging protocol and now routinely perform a full 10 minute acquisition over the epitrochlear region in any patient with a primary melanoma site on the forearm or hand. In this period we have found

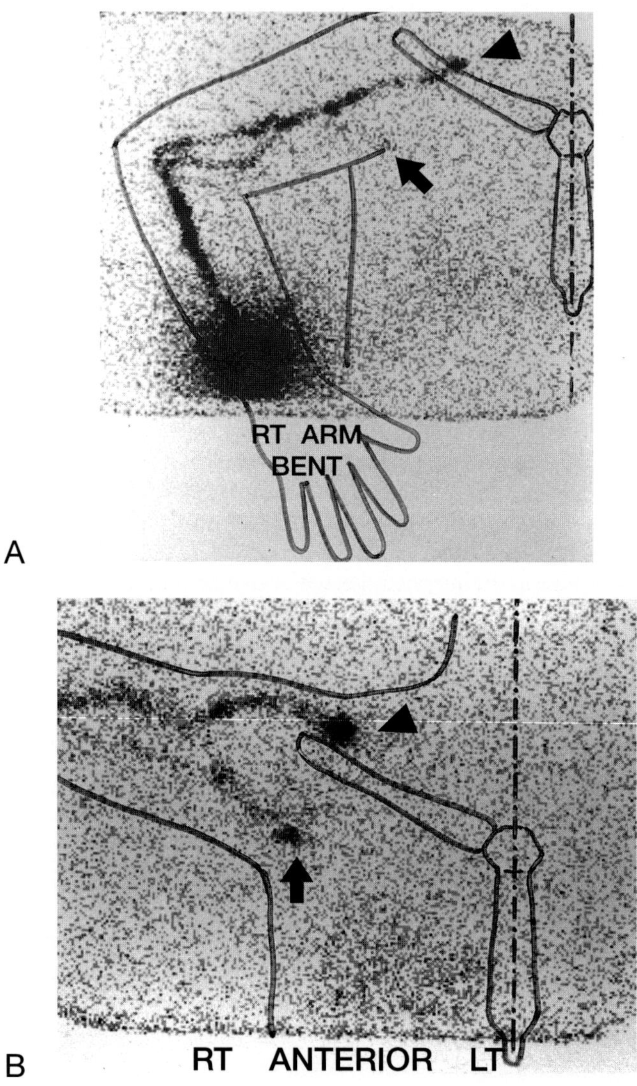

Figure 6.22 Drainage from the right wrist to the right axilla and right supraclavicular fossa

Dynamic scans (A and B) show 2 dominant lymphatic channels passing up the arm one to a node in the right axilla (arrow) and one to a node in the right supraclavicular fossa (arrowhead). These are both sentinel nodes.

drainage to the epitrochlear node group in 5 of 24 such patients which is an incidence of 21%. The implication of these data is that sentinel nodes in the epitrochlear region will be missed unless this area is carefully scanned in all patients with hand and forearm primary melanoma sites. The primary skin sites which drained to the epitrochlear nodes were on the medial and lateral dorsal and ventral skin surfaces of the forearm, the dorsum of the wrist and the back of the hand (Figure 4.7).

We have only once seen direct drainage from the skin of the forearm to an interpectoral or infraclavicular node.[101] As previously mentioned we have never seen direct drainage to the deltopectoral node group.

We have studied a total of 298 patients with primary melanoma sites on the upper limbs and shoulders (using a vertical line in a sagittal plane through the axilla to define the limits of the upper limb and shoulder versus the trunk). There were 206 patients with lesion sites on the anterior upper limb or shoulder and 92 with posterior lesion sites. The results in these patients are summarised in Table 6.5.

Of the 21 patients who had drainage to a sentinel node in the supraclavicular fossa there were 4 whose primary site was on the forearm.

6.4 LOWER LIMB

Conventional descriptions of the patterns of lymphatic drainage from the lower limb have been based largely on radiographic lymphography.[123, 124] These reports have described the lymphatic vessels of the lower limb as consisting of superficial (subcutaneous) prefascial and deep subfascial systems. The superficial system has anterior and posterior vessels. Injection on the dorsum of the foot, which is the usual site for lymphography, displays the anterior system and

Table 6.5 Upper limb primary sites

Draining node field	*Number of patients*	*% of total*
Axilla	289	97
Supraclavicular	21	7
Epitrochlear	11	4
Interpectoral	1	<1
Triangular intermuscular space	2	<1
Cervical Level V	1	<1
Interval nodes	14	5

usually does not cause opacification of the deep subfascial system. It is said that the medial side of the dorsum of the foot drains via anterior lymphatic vessels along the path of the long saphenous vein, while the lateral aspect of the dorsum of the foot drains via vessels which pass anteriorly and laterally below the knee. Lateral vessels tend towards the medial side of the leg just proximal to the knee[68], again following the long saphenous vein to the inguinal nodes. The lymphatics branch frequently and above the knee towards the groin there are often bifurcations. The posterior superficial system is displayed on lymphography by injecting a lymph vessel below the lateral malleolus. Clouse has stated that there are fewer lymph channels here and that they accompany the short saphenous vein to the popliteal fossa, where they enter the popliteal nodes.[68] From here efferent vessels turn anteromedially to become deep subfascial vessels and then pass with deep blood vessels on the medial aspect of the thigh to inguinal nodes. The deep subfascial system is not usually relevant in cutaneous lymphatic flow as valves direct flow from the deep to the superficial system and flow in the opposite direction is rare. As expected, lymphatic drainage from the lower limb is exclusively to the ipsilateral groin except when the patient has had prior surgery on the groin nodes and in this situation lymphatic channels may be seen passing across the pubis to contralateral groin nodes.

The above information about the lymphatic vessels of the leg has been derived almost exclusively from injections made into the dorsum of the foot. In lymphoscintigraphy, however, the site of injection of the tracer is determined by the site of the melanoma, thus we have observed lymphatic drainage from all parts of the skin of the lower limb. There is a general tendency for the lymph channels to pass medially, but there is a great variation in the path taken by these channels in different patients. Lymphatic channels from the leg commonly pass both medially and laterally up the lower limb. We have found that drainage to the popliteal nodes from the skin of the posterior leg or foot occurs in some patients who have primary sites on the dorsum of the foot, the sole of the heel, the medial heel and the lower calf on the medial side (Figure 4.9). This is a considerably more extensive distribution of sites than that suggested by Clouse, who found popliteal drainage only from the skin of the postero-lateral heel.

As is the case with drainage to the epitrochlear region, drainage to the popliteal fossa will be missed unless a full 10 minute acquisition is performed over this node field on delayed imaging. Relying on the presence of tracer in this area on the persistance scope is inadequate. Using this method we observed popliteal drainage in only 3 of 181 patients who had primary sites at or distal to the knee[125]. Over the last 15 months, however, we have been routinely acquiring a 10 minute image over the popliteal fossa in all patients with leg and foot primary melanoma sites. During this period we have seen drainage to the popliteal fossa in 8 of 50 such patients, an incidence of 16%. This suggests that with our original protocol we were not adequately documenting drainage to the popliteal fossa.

Channels from the leg branch frequently in the anterior thigh (Figure 5.1) and multiple sentinel nodes are the rule in the groin with lower limb injections rather than the exception.[103] The average number of sentinel nodes seen in the groin after lower limb injections is 3.3. It is quite common for channels to bypass nodes near the apex of the femoral triangle to drain directly into higher inguinal nodes (Figure 5.1).

Another consistent feature of lymphatic mapping in the lower limb is that second tier lymph nodes are frequently seen[86], often on the early dynamic phase component of the study. This is in contrast to the axilla where sentinel nodes are often the only nodes seen to contain tracer and even at 24 hours can remain the only significantly radioactive nodes.[85] The high incidence of second tier lymph nodes in the groin is associated with high lymph flow velocities, as noted earlier, and we have already mentioned that lymph flow rates from the lower limb are the highest seen in the skin[41] (see Figures 3.2 to 3.5).

We have now performed lymphatic mapping in 354 patients with primary sites on the lower limbs. There were 231 primary sites on the anterior lower limbs and 123 on the posterior lower limbs.

6.5 SCROTUM

We have performed lymphoscintigraphy following excision biopsy of melanomas of the scrotum in 2 patients. One was at the junction of scrotal and perineal skin on the right side and drained to right groin nodes. The second patient had a melanoma situated on the left side of the scrotum, and showed 4 dominant channels draining across the midline to 4 sentinel nodes in the right groin, plus a single lymph channel draining to a single sentinel node in the left groin. Drainage across the midline is thus possible from the skin of the scrotum. In the second patient an elective surgical dissection of the left groin would thus have missed four out of the five sentinel nodes.

Chapter 7

LYMPHATIC MAPPING OF THE BREAST

7.1 THE FIRST STUDIES

In the 1780s two investigators independently described lymphatic drainage from the breast to axillary and internal mammary nodes. These were Cruikshank in 1786[52] and Mascagni in 1787[54]. Both used mercury injected directly into the lymphatics of cadavers. Cruikshank thought that the nipple and more superficial breast tissue drained to the axilla while the deeper tissue drained to the internal mammary nodes via lymphatics which perforated the intercostal spaces. We no longer consider that this is correct. However, he also described intra-mammary interval nodes lying between the nipple and the axilla and mentioned that direct drainage could occur to nodes behind the middle of the clavicle. Thus Cruikshank all those years ago described several features of what we now regard as the lymphatic drainage of the breast. It is remarkable that both of these original studies emphasised the importance of drainage to the internal mammary nodes, yet for over 100 years this fact was essentially ignored in the management of patients with breast cancer. The first clinician to realise the importance of drainage to the internal mammary nodes was probably Handley, who after exploring the internal mammary nodes, found metastases in these nodes in some of his patients. Though he did not keep removing these nodes surgically on a routine basis, he did attempt to eliminate any possible metastases in them by inserting radium needles into the upper three intercostal spaces.[126]

7.2 ONE HUNDRED YEARS LATER

Almost 100 years after the original studies of Cruikshank and Mascagni, Sappey described what he regarded as two discrete lymphatic drainage systems for the breast. These were superficial lymphatics which drained the skin over the breast and deep lymphatics which drained the mammary gland itself. Sappey said that the two systems showed frequent anastomoses[15], and that the superficial lymphatic vessels draining the skin over the breast invariably drained to the axilla, as illustrated in Figure 2.3. Sappey described the lymphatic drainage of the mammary gland itself as originating in the tissues surrounding the mammary lobules and then passing via collecting vessels in a central direction with the mammary ducts towards the nipple. He thought that all of these collecting vessels emptied into a subareolar lymphatic plexus from which two large collecting vessels passed to the axilla, one arising from the medial aspect of the subareolar plexus and one from the lateral aspect. Later Rouviere described similar findings but these studies appear to have been performed on the cadavers of infants and these two dominant channels do not seem to be a major feature in the lymphatic drainage of the adult breast.[121] As mentioned later, it is possible that accidental injection into a mammary duct caused the accumulation of mercury into the subareolar region (see section 7.5 and Chapter 10).

Using blue dye Gerota showed multiple possible routes of lymphatic drainage from the breast[60], and surgical practice confirmed that metastases from breast cancer could occur in several different lymph node groups. Rotter while studying excised specimens of breast cancer showed lymphatics passing from the posterior aspect of the breast through the pectoralis major muscle to interpectoral nodes.[127] About a third of the cases he studied showed metastases in these nodes. This information led to the recommendation that both pectoral muscles be removed during radical mastectomy for breast cancer.

7.3 BREAST LYMPHANGIOGRAPHY

In the 1960s several researchers began using lymphangiography to study the lymphatic drainage of the breast and demonstrated variable patterns of drainage.[128–130] They attempted to use the test to diagnose metastases and claimed some success, though most surgeons did not find the test sufficiently accurate to be useful in this role.

7.4 THE CLEARING TECHNIQUE TO EXAMINE DRAINING NODE FIELDS

Another useful method of studying the lymphatic drainage of the breast was to carefully examine surgical specimens following axillary dissection using the clearing technique.[131] The method relies on dissolving the fat so that the specimen becomes translucent which allows small lymph nodes to be seen which might otherwise have been missed. This allowed the frequency of metastasis in the various axillary node groups to be compared to the site of the primary tumour in the breast but of course gave no information on drainage to other node fields unless these too had been excised. Using this technique Haagensen and colleagues showed that the central group of nodes in the axilla was involved in 90% of patients with metastases.[66] The axillary vein group of nodes was involved in 33.8% of the patients with nodal metastases and the external mammary group of nodes was involved in only 7.5% of them. By this time radiocolloids had also been used to map the pattern of lymph drainage from the breast.

7.5 EARLY RADIOCOLLOID LYMPHATIC MAPPING OF THE BREAST

The first radiocolloid to be used to map the lymphatic drainage of the breast was colloidal gold-198. Hultborn and colleagues injected this radiocolloid into the breast prior to radical mastectomy and then studied the radioactivity in the specimen and the patient.[132] They showed that the movement of tracer from the breast was mostly to the axilla (97–99%) with only a small amount passing to the internal mammary nodes (1–3%). Turner-Warwick, again using colloidal gold-198, injected the breast prior to radical mastectomy and then used autoradiographs to detect lymph drainage to the axillary and internal mammary nodes.[133] He found that the ipsilateral axillary and internal mammary chains could receive drainage from any quadrant of the breast. He demonstrated that the subareolar plexus as described by Sappey and later by Rouviere was not an important pathway for the lymphatic drainage of the breast. In fact Turner-Warwick speculated that the description of the movement of vital dyes and/or mercury to the subareolar region was caused by direct injection of the milk ducts and not lymphatic drainage to this area. He also showed that lymphatic vessels passed through the substance of the breast tissue to the draining node fields and did not lie only on the anterior or posterior surface of the mammary tissue as had previously been thought. The lymphatic drainage from the four quadrants of the breast was studied by Vendrell-Torne and colleagues in 1972 using colloidal gold-198.[134] They showed that the patterns of lymphatic drainage from the breast varied when different breast quadrants were injected with tracer. Many workers have since confirmed these findings. The tracer used in these original studies (colloidal gold-198) emits beta particles and thus delivers a significant radiation dose to breast tissue. For this reason it is not used today and 99mTc labelled colloidal agents are preferred.

7.6 THE NEXT PHASE OF LYMPHOSCINTIGRAPHY IN BREAST CANCER

Over the next 20 years, lymphatic mapping in patients with breast cancer focused on one of two strategies, neither of which actually mapped the lymphatic drainage of the breast cancer itself. The first strategy aimed at determining if lymph nodes draining the breast of patients with breast cancer contained metastatic deposits. The three techniques used in this endeavour were axillary lymphoscintigraphy, mammary lymphoscintigraphy and internal mammary lymphoscintigraphy.

The second strategy was to show the location of internal mammary nodes using internal mammary lymphoscintigraphy to aid in radiation treatment planning. These strategies met with varying success.

7.6.1 Lymphatic Mapping Intended to Diagnose Nodal Metastases

7.6.1.1 *Axillary lymphoscintigraphy (AxLS)*

Axillary lymphoscintigraphy (AxLS) involved the interdigital injection of radiocolloid in the hand to image the axillary lymph nodes.[135] The studies were then evaluated for the presence of metastatic deposits in the nodes. Both hands were injected and nodes showing decreased or irregular uptake were considered to contain metastases. The symmetry of uptake in one axilla versus the opposite side was also considered an important factor in interpretation. AxLS was also used sometimes to check the axilla intra-operatively[136] or post-operatively[137] to confirm that an adequate axillary lymph node dissection had been performed. However, it never became popular in this role. The technique of AxLS was not found to be an accurate method of staging the axilla for metastases and is no longer used for this purpose.

7.6.1.2 *Mammary lymphoscintigraphy (MLS)*

The search for a method of diagnosing the presence of metastases in the draining lymph nodes of patients with breast cancer was pursued further using the technique of mammary lymphoscintigraphy. A variety of approaches was taken, including the following.

- Intratumoral injection

In 1981 Gabelle and colleagues studied 100 patients with breast cancer after intratumoral injection of 99mTc-labelled colloidal rhenium, a colloid that has a favourable particle size distribution for lymphoscintigraphy.[138] The number of nodes seen on delayed scans 1 to 4 hours later was noted and compared with the histological findings in the nodes after axillary lymphadenectomy. Patients with more than 3 metastatic axillary nodes had on average 2 or less lymph nodes visualised on lymphoscintigraphy while patients with less than 3 metastatic lymph nodes had more than 2 nodes visualised on scan. This difference in groups was highly significant. However, the results were not useful in clinical decision making in individual patients.

Serin and colleagues scanned 51 patients after preoperative intratumoral injection of 2.5 mCi of 99mTc antimony sulphide colloid to determine the accuracy of MLS in diagnosing nodal metastases.[139] They compared the scans with clinical examination of the axilla preoperatively and with nodal histology after surgical removal of the axillary nodes. They found MLS of no value in diagnosing axillary lymph node metastases and concluded that it was less accurate than clinical examination in diagnosing axillary metastases.

- Periareolar injection

Gasparini and colleagues used periareolar injection of 99mTc sulphur colloid in 26 patients with breast cancer.[140] Scans were performed in the search for metastases. The number of nodes visualised in the axilla was compared to pathology. They noted 2 of 26 patients had more than 3 nodes visualised in the axilla but felt that no useful data were obtained with the technique.

- Subareolar injection

The above technique was modified by Mazzeo and coworkers, who administered subareolar injections of 99mTc albumin nanocolloid in 32 patients and scanned the axilla for metastases.[141] They too compared the number of nodes visualised on lymphoscintigraphy with pathological findings after surgical removal of the nodes. They demonstrated nodes in the axilla in 87.5% of patients but the method was unable to reliably diagnose the presence of axillary lymph node metastases.

- Periosteal injection of the ribs

Terui and Yamamoto studied 100 patients with breast cancer using bilateral sub-periosteal injections of 99mTc rhenium colloid.[142] They demonstrated internal mammary nodes on the side of the cancer in 91% of patients and on the opposite side in 93%. Axillary nodes were demonstrated on the side of the cancer in 85% and on the normal side in 86%. No data were presented to show that this approach could diagnose nodal metastases. Furthermore, the lymph nodes visualised would have been nodes receiving drainage from the ribs not the breast tissue. This approach has not been pursued by others.

- Intradermal injection

Matsubara and colleagues used intradermal injections of 99mTc rhenium colloid around the surgical wound in 64 patients following surgical removal of a breast cancer.[143] Contralateral axillary nodes were often visualised, as well as nodes in the ipsilateral axilla. These data seem of doubtful relevance to the breast tumor lymphatic drainage, as the method was clearly evaluating dermal lymphatic drainage not the breast lymphatics. Dermal lymphatic pathways are also likely to have been altered significantly in these patients by the prior surgery on the breast. There have been occasional suggestions that the intradermal injection of radiocolloid in the skin overlying a breast cancer may be an easy way of finding the sentinel node in the axilla. We strongly disagree with this concept as the lymphatic channels which drain breast tissue are undoubtedly different from those draining the skin over the breast. This is illustrated by the fact that inner quadrant breast tissue often drains to the internal mammary node chain while the skin over the inner quadrant of the breast never does. Breast tissue and the skin over the breast clearly have discrete lymphatic drainage systems and intradermal injections will not define sentinel nodes draining intramammary breast cancers.

- Intramammary injection

Saeki and colleagues studied 12 patients with breast tumours and injected 99mTc labelled activated carbon microspheres into the breast tissue at unspecified locations.[144] They observed tracer in axillary, subclavian or parasternal lymph nodes in 10 patients 1 hour after injection. No comment was made on whether the visualised lymph nodes appeared normal or otherwise.

None of these methods was clinically useful in diagnosing axillary lymph node metastases and none was widely adopted, though there were pockets of enthusiasm for several of these approaches. This strategy of trying to use lymphoscintigraphy to diagnose the presence of metastases in lymph nodes was never likely to succeed due to the poor spatial resolution of lymphoscintigraphic studies.

7.6.1.3 *Internal mammary lymphoscintigraphy (IMLS)*

Described by Rossi[145] in 1966 and shortly afterwards by Schenck[146], internal mammary lymphoscintigraphy (IMLS) was developed later by Gunes Ege at the Princess Margaret Hospital in Toronto.[147] The method involved injection of radiocolloid into the space between the anterior and posterior rectus sheaths in the upper abdomen and then imaging the tracer as it passed upwards via the internal mammary lymph node chain. The initial studies using IMLS were again performed to evaluate the internal mammary lymph node chain for the presence of metastases in patients with breast cancer. Images were interpreted as being normal or suggesting metastatic involvement of the nodes. Scan features which were thought to indicate metastatic involvement included: decreased activity in individual nodes, visualisation of few lower parasternal nodes because of obstruction to distal flow, or obvious asymmetry in internal mammary node uptake in one chain versus the opposite side. Though several studies which showed promising results using this technique to diagnose metastases were published[148, 149] and many authors suggested a significant role for IMLS in the management of patients with breast cancer[150–154] it never became widely used and is now rarely performed.

This approach to lymphatic mapping of the breast was not using the strengths of LS, that is its ability to accurately map physiological lymphatic drainage. Lymphoscintigraphy has high physiological resolution but low spatial resolution. Instead, these studies had focused attention on the major limitation of LS, namely its poor spatial resolution. Lymphoscintigraphy using conventional radiocolloids is not likely to be able to diagnose the presence of micrometastases in lymph nodes, just as radiographic lymphangiography proved inadequate in this role. However, if labelled antibodies to specific tumour antigens can be developed, then this objective may be achieved in the future.

7.6.2 Lymphatic Mapping to Locate Internal Mammary Nodes for Radiation Therapy

The second strategy used over this interim period was to display and mark the location of the internal mammary lymph node chain as an aid to radiation therapy planning in patients with breast cancer, using the technique of internal mammary lymphoscintigraphy. Many investigators used the technique in this way.[155–158] In this role IMLS proved reasonably successful, with a significant percentage of internal mammary nodes being identified which would not have been included in a standard radiation therapy field of this node chain. It is still used for this purpose in some centres.

Chapter 8

THE SENTINEL NODE CONCEPT IN BREAST CANCER

To this point lymphatic mapping in the breast had essentially been used in patients with breast cancer in an attempt to diagnose the presence of metastases in draining lymph nodes or to locate the internal mammary nodes for radiation therapy. AxLS, MLS and IMLS had all been used in this way. IMLS had also been used with some success to locate the internal mammary nodes in three dimensions to ensure that all nodes were included in radiation therapy fields. However, the whole thrust of lymphatic mapping in patients with breast cancer changed after Morton and colleagues described the concept of the sentinel lymph node in melanoma. The aim of lymphatic mapping in the breast using radiocolloids then became to locate the sentinel lymph node prior to surgical biopsy.

Following the finding by Morton and colleagues in 1992 that a lymph node field in patients with melanoma could be accurately staged by surgically removing only the sentinel lymph node or nodes, interest quickly developed in determining if this also held true in patients with breast cancer.[104] It is logical of course that the sentinel node concept in breast cancer should be identical to that in melanoma, i.e. to locate and remove all sentinel nodes draining the primary tumour site. It is therefore interesting that this is not what many workers have done when approaching the sentinel nodes in breast cancer patients. Most groups have concentrated only on the axilla and have not looked for or have ignored sentinel nodes occurring in the internal mammary or supraclavicular node fields — the two other node fields which drain the breast.

8.1 THE RATIONALE FOR AXILLARY NODE STAGING

It remains true that the single best prognostic factor in patients with breast cancer is the histological status of their axillary lymph nodes.[159, 160] Even in patients with breast cancers confined to the inner quadrants of the breast, metastatic involvement of the axilla is more likely than metastatic involvement of the internal mammary chain (42% versus 28%).[161] The status of the axillary nodes is therefore considered important in planning therapeutic strategies using adjuvant chemotherapy. If no axillary nodes are removed there is a roughly 50% incidence of disease recurrence here in patients without clinically involved nodes on presentation.[159] Axillary node sampling thus offers potential benefits in the control of locoregional recurrence.

8.2 THE RATIONALE FOR SENTINEL NODE BIOPSY OF THE AXILLA

Patients have for some time been routinely subjected to an elective dissection of the axillary lymph nodes on the side of the breast cancer to determine the nodal status of the axilla, with considerable associated morbidity including scarring, numbness and lymphoedema. In breast cancer patients with no clinically suspicious axillary lymph nodes about 40% overall will have microscopic metastases found at operation.[162] The size of the tumour is the only accurate predictor of axillary involvement with metastasis in cancer of the breast, and there is a direct correlation between the size of the primary tumour and the incidence of nodal metastases.[163] Tumours less than 1 cm in diameter showed 13% positive nodes while tumours greater than 1 cm in diameter had 30% positive nodes. Population screening with mammography means that more patients today are being found with these smaller lesions, thus the majority of patients who now present with breast cancer will not harbour metastases in the axillary nodes. These patients will not accrue any benefit from axillary lymphadenectomy. If a selective sampling of 1 or 2 sentinel nodes could accurately stage the axillary node field this would be a significant advance as it would avoid unnecessary surgery in this majority of patients who have no nodal metastases. On the other hand patients who had a positive sentinel node could then proceed to an elective axillary lymphadenectomy to fully stage the axillary nodes and remove any further involved nodes, while those patients with a negative sentinel node could avoid further unnecessary surgery. The results of sentinel node biopsy could also be used to select patients for adjuvant therapy protocols.

In patients who had elective axillary node dissections there was a variable incidence of 'skip' metastases in Level II or III nodes. It is likely that these were simply the sentinel nodes located at Level II or III.

8.3 SUCCESSFUL SENTINEL NODE BIOPSY OF THE AXILLA

Krag accurately located the sentinel lymph node in the axilla of 18 of 22 patients who had received peritumoral injections of radiocolloid preoperatively.[164] Seven of 7 patients with proven metastases were identified and in 3 of them the sentinel node was the only positive node.

Giuliano and colleagues documented the accuracy of the original blue dye method in locating the sentinel node in breast cancer patients and in the latter part of their study a sentinel node in the axilla was found in 78% of their patients.[165] The overall sensitivity of the sentinel node biopsy technique was 88% with a specificity of 100%. They improved their results with experience and in the last half of the study there were no false negative sentinel nodes.

8.4 MORE THAN JUST AXILLARY DRAINAGE

Uren and colleagues showed that peritumoral injections of 99mTc antimony sulphide colloid allowed the pattern of lymphatic drainage for individual breast cancers to be determined in over 90% of patients.[166] They demonstrated drainage across the centre line of the breast to internal mammary or axillary nodes in 32% of patients with outer and inner quadrant tumours respectively. Upper quadrant lesions drained directly to supraclavicular nodes in 20% of patients, and in 85% of all patients drainage occurred to the ipsilateral axilla. In the 3 patients who had the sentinel node removed with the aid of blue dye injection preoperatively it was negative in 1 patient who had no metastases in other nodes (0/11 nodes) and positive in the other 2 patients, both of whom did have metastases in other nodes (2/23 and 8/14 nodes).

8.5 ACCURACY CONFIRMED

Subsequent studies have confirmed the accuracy of sentinel node biopsy in the axilla for patients with breast cancer.[77, 163, 167] Albertini and colleagues, using a combination of blue dye and an intraoperative gamma detection probe after peritumoral injection of tracer, identified a sentinel node in 92% of their 62 patients and 32% of patients had a sentinel node positive for metastases.[77] There were no false negative sentinel nodes. In 67% of their patients with positive nodes the sentinel nodes were the only positive nodes. These authors pointed out, as others have done, another advantage of the sentinel node biopsy approach, i.e. when the histopathologist is given only one or two sentinel nodes to examine he/she can examine these much more carefully than he/she would be able to examine a radical dissection specimen of the axilla. Special techniques such as serial sectioning, immunohistochemical staining[168] and reverse transcriptase-polymerase chain reaction analysis[169] may also be applied to improve the sensitivity of detecting micrometastases in sentinel nodes.

8.6 SENTINEL NODE BIOPSY USING A GAMMA PROBE WITHOUT LYMPHOSCINTIGRAPHY IN BREAST CANCER

As the possible patterns of lymphatic drainage from the breast are simpler than those of the skin, some have suggested that lymphoscintigraphy using a high resolution gamma camera is not necessary when performing selective sentinel node biopsy of the axilla in patients with breast cancer. Some researchers argue that a gamma detecting probe alone is adequate to accurately locate and remove the sentinel node in the axilla.[164] Usually radiocolloid is injected into the breast around the tumour prior to surgery. The delay between injection and surgery varies but is usually between 20 minutes and 3 hours. The gamma probe is used to 'scan' the axilla in a crude rectilinear fashion to locate the radioactive sentinel node. A small skin incision is then made and the node found using the gamma probe to guide the surgeon to the 'hot' node. When the 'hot' sentinel node has been removed the axillary node field should then record only background counts on the gamma probe. Since most patients with breast cancer will have a single sentinel node in the axilla[166] there is a certain attraction to the idea that a simplified sentinel node biopsy procedure will be adequate in breast cancer patients. Not performing high resolution lymphoscintigraphy will also decrease the cost of the sentinel node biopsy procedure.

Though this has been reported to be an accurate method of locating and removing the axillary sentinel node, we believe there remain several problems with this approach.[110] The method will fail if there has been no migration of tracer from the injection sites to the axilla. The speed of movement of tracer to the draining node fields varies from patient to patient. If lymphoscintigraphy has been performed this problem can be detected and further more vigorous massage of the injection site can be performed to ensure movement of the tracer to the sentinel node, prior to any attempt at surgical biopsy.

The lack of a high resolution image will also mean that intramammary interval nodes are likely to be missed. These are often near the injection site and will not be detectable using a probe due to scattered radiation from the primary site (Figure 8.1). Such interval nodes are by definition sentinel nodes and should be removed if the sentinel node biopsy procedure is to be successful.

A further problem with using a gamma probe without lymphoscintigraphy is that not all radioactive nodes are sentinel nodes. In some patients second tier lymph nodes are seen in the axilla. These are nodes which have received tracer which has already passed through the filter function of a sentinel node. Removing all radioactive nodes in such a patient will thus entail the unnecessary removal of second tier lymph nodes. Though some will argue that using large particle colloids tends to decrease the amount of tracer in second tier nodes and thus obviates this difficulty such an approach produces its own problems, as large particle colloids do not accurately map the physiology of the lymphatic system.

Sentinel nodes will be missed if this strategy is followed. As well, any radiocolloid has a range of particle sizes and even the so-called large particle colloids such as 99mTc sulphur colloid will show second tier nodes in some patients. There is good evidence that this is occurring. Gulec and colleagues[176] found some patients with 5 and 6 sentinel nodes in the axilla using 99mTc sulphur colloid, while using 99mTc antimony sulphide colloid we have only ever seen 1 patient with more than 2 axillary sentinel nodes (see Chapter 10.13).

High resolution lymphoscintigraphy also allows sentinel nodes in the supraclavicular fossa and the internal mammary lymph node chains to be located and marked. Studies with a probe alone have found that scattered radiation from the injection site has made location of the internal mammary nodes impossible and such studies have not mentioned any attempt to locate supraclavicular nodes. If lymphatic drainage to the internal mammary and or supraclavicular lymph nodes is detected on lymphoscintigraphy, it is logical that these sentinel nodes should be removed along with any axillary sentinel node if the sentinel node biopsy procedure is to be complete.[170] Not removing all sentinel nodes means an incomplete sentinel node biopsy procedure. Though many do not currently look for or remove sentinel nodes outside the axilla we believe this is important and will prove to be a major limitation of the gamma probe only method of sentinel node biopsy in breast cancer.

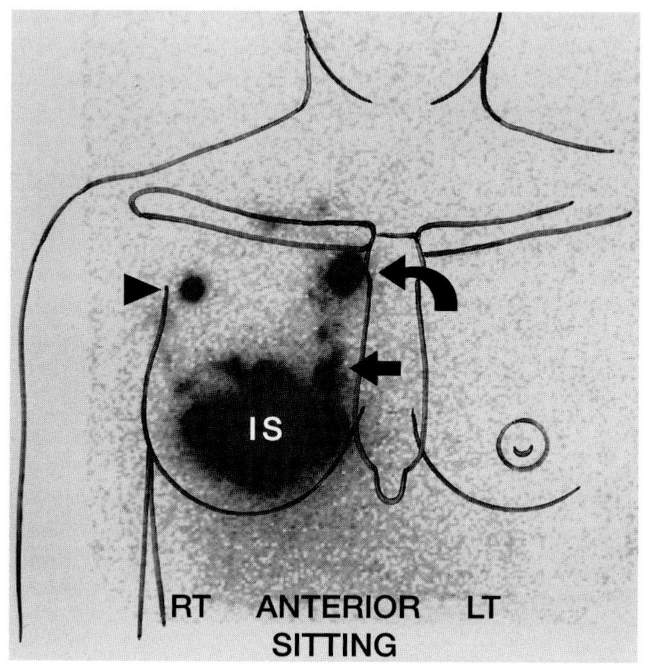

A

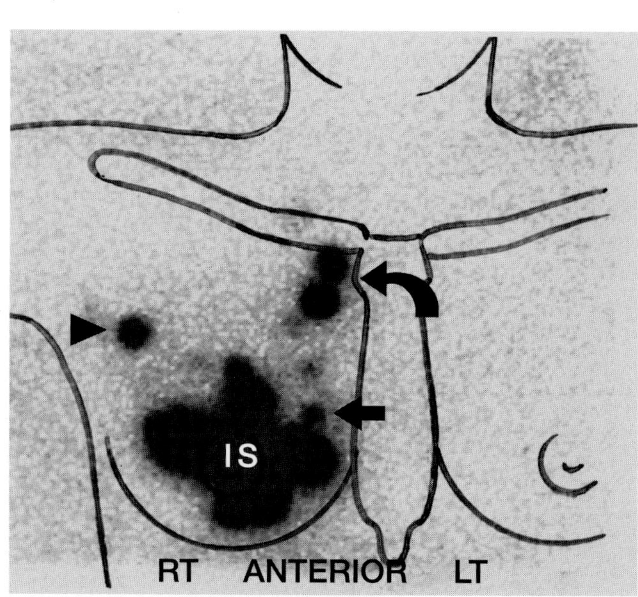

B

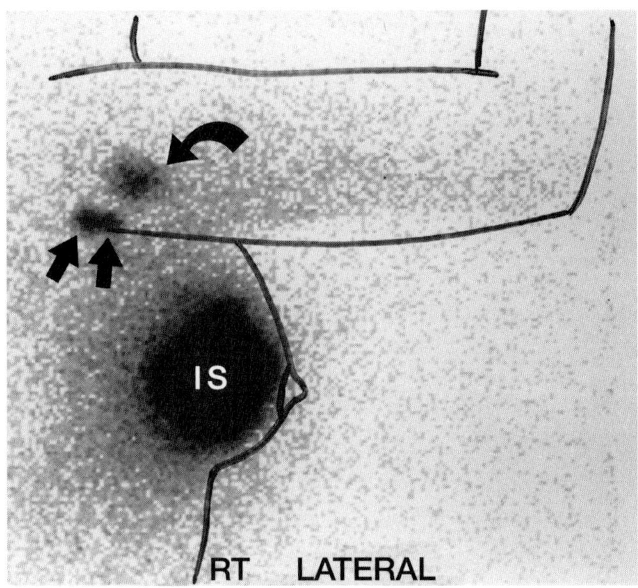

Figure 8.1 Drainage to an intramammary interval node

A: Tracer has been injected (IS) around the primary tumour in the RUIQ adjacent to the areola. In the early dynamic phase a curving channel is seen passing towards the right axilla where there appears to be a single sentinel node (arrowhead). There is also activity in an interval node in the medial aspect of the breast above the injection sites (arrow) and tracer in 2 sentinel nodes in the upper right internal mammary chain (curved arrow). The activity in the intramammary interval node would not be found without lymphoscintigraphy as a gamma probe alone would be swamped by scattered counts from the nearby injection sites. B: Delayed scan in the anterior projection confirms these findings. C: Right lateral scan shows that there are actually 2 right axillary sentinel nodes lying one in front of the other (arrows). This shows the importance of lateral views of the axilla to confirm the number of sentinel nodes. The upper internal mamary sentinel nodes are also faintly seen (curved arrow).

Chapter 9

MAMMARY LYMPHOSCINTIGRAPHY

9.1 LOCATING THE BREAST CANCER

Our technique is to use high resolution ultrasound to accurately locate the primary breast tumour. All but one of our cases were clinically palpable and the impalpable lesion was visible on ultrasound. The ultrasound is performed with the patient in the position to be used for injection of the radiopharmaceutical. The size of the tumour and its depth from the skin is recorded. The distance from the skin to the centre of the tumour is measured.

9.2 INJECTING THE TRACER

A hole is cut in an incontinence sheet and this is placed over the breast to isolate the area to be injected. This is to avoid contamination of the skin with any spilled isotope. The skin is cleaned with iodine solution and 4 injections of tracer are given around the tumour at the depth of the centre of the tumour. These are placed at 12, 3, 6 and 9 o'clock around the tumour. We use 1 ml syringes with 5–10 MBq of 99mTc-antimony sulphide colloid solution in a volume of 0.2 ml for each injection. A slightly larger volume of injectate is used in the breast compared to the skin in the hope of increasing interstitial pressure and thus facilitating entry of the tracer into the lymphatic capillaries. We have noticed that there is much less resistance to injection in breast tissue compared to skin and have recently increased the volume of tracer injected from 0.1 to 0.2 ml for breast lymphoscintigraphy. This is to more closely approximate the interstitial pressures achieved in the skin following intradermal injection of tracer. We still believe, however, that higher volumes of injectate may be non-physiological and cause the visualisation of lymph channels and nodes which do not actually drain the breast cancer site.

The aim is to place the injection in normal breast tissue immediately adjacent to the tumour and not to inject the tumour itself (Figure 9.1). Long bore 25 gauge needles are used. After injecting the patient, a sterile pad is placed over the injection site and the patient is asked to perform gentle massage over the tumour in a rotary fashion for 5 minutes using the opposite hand.

9.3 IMAGING THE PATIENT

An early image is obtained over 10 minutes to identify any early dominant channels. If channels are seen passing to the axilla on these early scans, a lateral image is acquired to determine if there is more than one sentinel node in the axilla (see Figure 8.1). The patient then ambulates and moves the arms

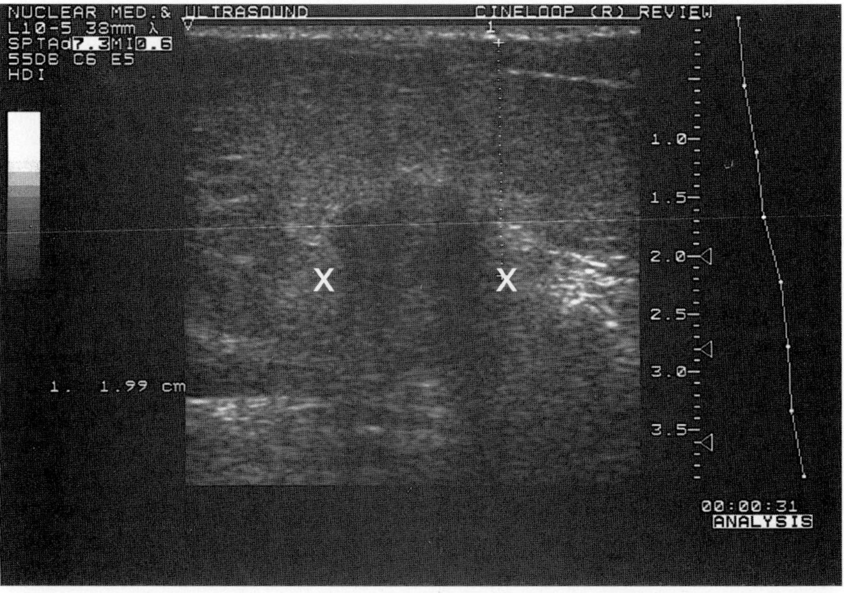

Figure 9.1 Site of injection for mammary lymphoscintigraphy

This ultrasound examination of a breast cancer was performed using a high resolution 5–10 MHz probe on an ATL Ultramark 9 HDI machine. The depth of the cancer from the skin has been measured at just under 2 cm and the four injections are given around the tumour at the 12, 3, 6, and 9 o'clock positions at the depth of the centre of the tumour. The tracer is injected into the normal breast tissue immediately adjacent to the cancer (white crosses).

normally until delayed scans are performed. These delayed scans are performed 2 to 3 hours after injection of the tracer. An anterior image is obtained with and without a transmission source behind the patient. The study without a transmission source is important as sometimes the sentinel nodes are quite faint and will be obscured by activity from an external source. A lateral view of the axilla is also routinely performed at this time, as sentinel nodes in the axilla are often obscured by the injection site in the anterior view. This is especially so for tumours in the upper outer quadrant, which is the most common site for primary breast cancer. We sometimes find it advantageous to acquire images with the patient sitting upright. This is particularly useful if the patient has pendulous breasts, as these will tend to fall laterally into the axilla when the patient is supine thus obscuring axillary nodes, but will hang down away from the axilla when the patient is upright (Figure 9.2).

9.4 MARKING THE SENTINEL NODES

After the delayed imaging is complete the sentinel nodes are marked. We mark the surface location of each node with a small tattoo of carbon black ink and a cross of Castellani's paint with the patient in the exact position to be used at surgery. We also measure the depth of the node from the skin with the patient in this position. This is achieved by placing a small amount of tracer in a needle hub on the skin at the site of the cross in the axilla and then imaging in the anterior projection. The distance between the node and the skin mark can then be measured directly from the film. The surface location of sentinel nodes in the internal mammary and supraclavicular node fields is also marked. The depth of supraclavicular nodes can be measured but activity at the injection site usually prevents this measurement for internal mammary nodes. This is less important because the anatomical location of the internal mammary nodes is quite consistent even though the depth of the nodes from the skin surface will vary between patients.

On completion of the study the patient leaves the department with the films and the report. Surgery is performed later the same day or the next day. There usually remain adequate counts in the sentinel nodes for up to 24 hours to allow their detection using an intraoperative gamma detecting probe. This approach also obviates the need to use radioisotopes in the operating theatre suite and greatly lessens radiation safety issues for theatre staff. A further advantage of performing surgery between 6 and 24 hours after tracer injection is that tracer has washed out of the soft tissues around the sentinel nodes, which increases the target to background ratio when using a gamma probe.

A

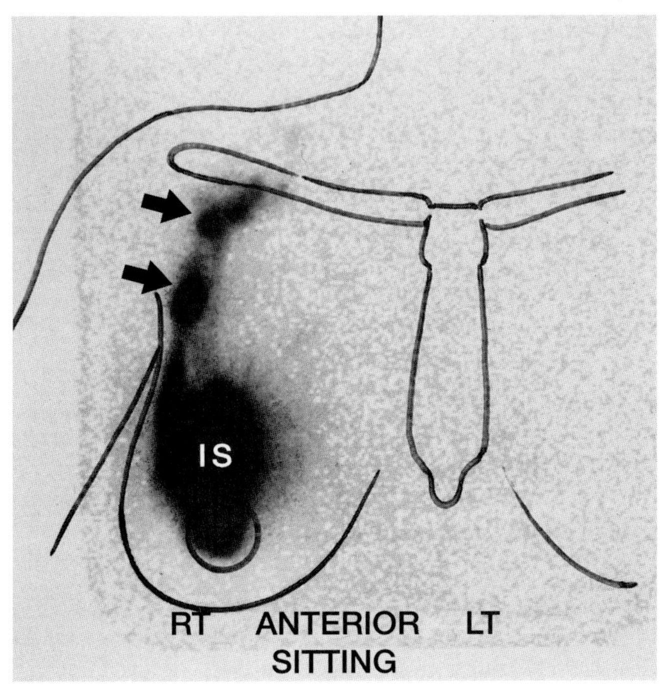

B

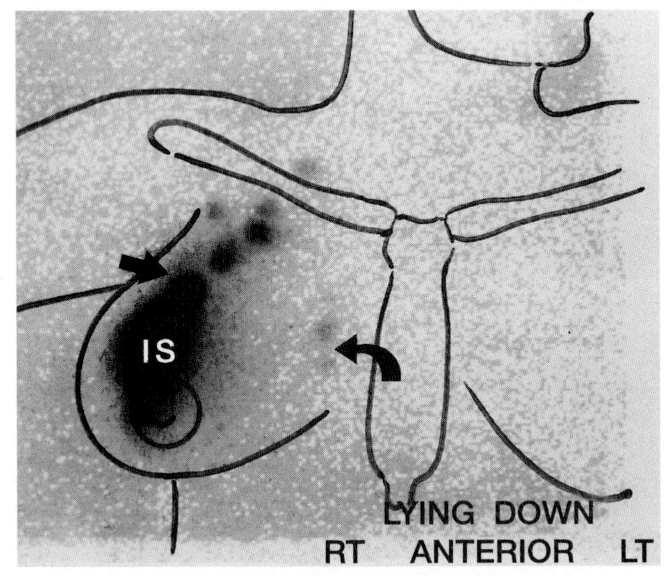

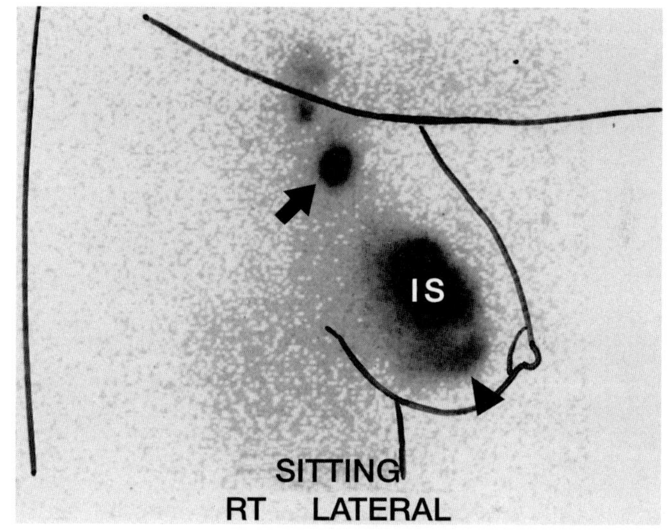

C

Figure 9.2 A pendulous breast may hide an axillary sentinel node

A: Dynamic breast lymphoscintigraphy performed in the sitting position facing the gamma camera in a patient with a right upper outer quadrant cancer. The injection sites (IS) bloom to a single area. Two channels are seen passing towards the right axilla, one to a sentinel node low in the axilla and one to a higher sentinel node. The pendulous breast in this patient falls down away from the axilla so that both sentinel nodes are clearly seen (arrows). B: The delayed scan in the anterior projection with the patient supine shows that the breast has fallen into the axillary area and the lowest sentinel node (arrow) is now partially obscured by the activity in the injection sites (IS). Faint activity is seen in 2 internal mammary nodes (curved arrow). C: In the delayed lateral view again with the patient sitting the first of the sentinel nodes (arrow) is seen clearly separate from the injection sites (IS). Some tracer has been injected into a mammary duct (arrowhead) and passes toward the nipple.

Chapter 10

PATTERNS OF LYMPHATIC DRAINAGE IN BREAST CANCER

We have performed lymphatic mapping using lymphoscintigraphy in over 150 patients with breast cancer. This chapter is an analysis of our first 102 patients, 99 females and 3 males. The location of the primary tumours is illustrated in Figure 10.1. Ten patients showed no movement of the tracer from the injection sites around the cancer. Since we introduced post-injection massage over the injection sites in late 1997, this phenomenon has become rare and has only occurred in 2 patients, 1 of whom had clinically palpable involved nodes in the axilla and the other who had a 3 cm metastatic intramammary node lying between the cancer in the right upper outer quadrant and the right axilla. It is likely therefore that the lymphatic channels were blocked by tumour in these patients.

Lymphatic drainage in our patients has occurred via lymph vessels which passed directly through the breast tissue to the draining node fields. We have not seen drainage via the so-called sub-areolar plexus. In 5–10% of patients, however, we have seen some tracer which has inadvertently been injected into a milk duct, pass anteriorly to the nipple area (see Figure 9.2). We suspect, as Turner-Warwick did,[133] that this phenomenon has been mistaken for drainage to a sub-areolar plexus by some previous researchers.

10.1 DRAINING NODE FIELDS PER PATIENT

In the 92 patients in whom we obtained a map of lymphatic drainage there were 52 patients who showed drainage to 1 node field, 34 who showed drainage to 2 node fields and 6 patients who showed drainage to all 3 node fields which drain breast tissue. Thus, 43% of our patients who showed lymph drainage of the tracer had multiple draining node fields. This number is important as it implies that in 2 of every 5 patients, sentinel node biopsy of only one node field will provide incomplete information. If about one third of draining nodes contain metastases then positive nodes will be missed in about 14% of patients.

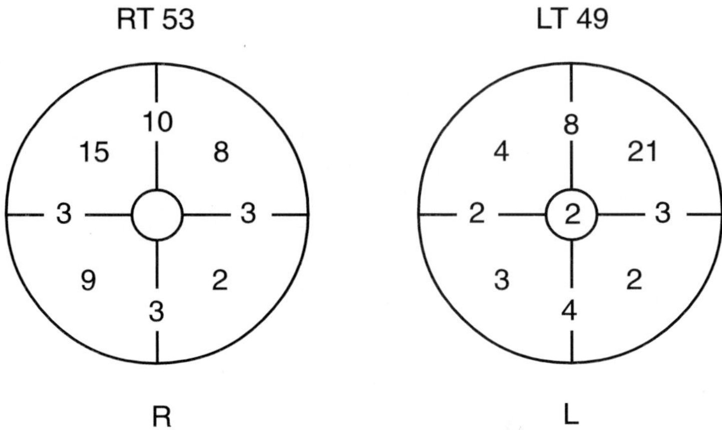

Figure 10.1 The location of the primary breast cancers

10.2 AXILLARY DRAINAGE DOMINATES

In 85 of the 92 patients (92%) the pattern of drainage included the axilla. This finding is in accord with the many previous studies which have been performed on the lymphatic drainage of the breast. It is also in accord with the clinical observation that metastases from breast cancer usually involve the axilla and that removal of axillary metastases can sometimes lead to cure of the disease. Drainage to the ipsilateral axilla can occur from any quadrant of the breast and it is known that metastases to the axilla occur regularly from primaries in all quadrants of the breast (Figure 10.2), though it is true that upper outer quadrant primaries show the highest incidence of axillary metastases.[66] In our patients who showed any drainage at all, 32 of 33 (97%) with upper outer quadrant lesions included drainage to the ipsilateral axilla. For cancers in the lower outer quadrant 11 of 11 patients (100%) included axillary drainage, while for the lower inner quadrant 3 of 4 (75%) included axillary drainage. For the upper inner quadrant the figure was 7 of 9 patients (78%). Many of our patients had cancers which lay at the junction of 2 breast quadrants. In patients with cancers totally in the outer half of the breast 48 of 49 (98%) included axillary drainage, while with wholely inner quadrant lesions 13 of 18 (72%) included axillary drainage.

10.3 INTERNAL MAMMARY DRAINAGE

Of the 18 patients with lesions in the inner quadrants of the breast and who showed drainage of the radiocolloid to lymph nodes, 14 (78%) included internal

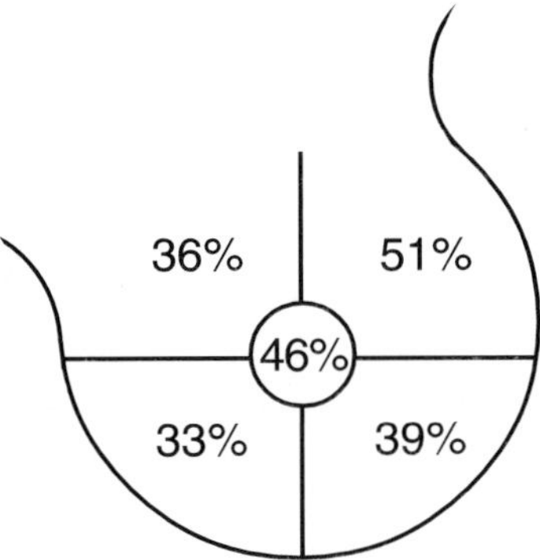

Figure 10.2 The incidence of axillary metastases from the different breast quadrants

Source: Adapted from Haagensen, C.D., Feind, C.R., Herter, F.P., Slanetz, C.A. and Weinberg, J.A. (1972) *The Lymphatics in Cancer*, p. 583. Philadelphia: W. B. Saunders Co.

mammary drainage. Four other patients with inner quadrant primaries had no migration of the tracer. In the 49 patients with wholely outer quadrant lesions 17 (35%) included internal mammary drainage. In our patients who showed drainage to the internal mammary node field this most often seemed to occur to a node in about the 3rd interspace, and it was not uncommon to see one or two more nodes above the presumed sentinel node in the internal mammary chain. Drainage to these nodes often seemed to occur via a curvilinear channel which passed from the medial aspect of the breast just below the level of the areola (Figure 10.3). There are usually about 9 internal mammary nodes in each patient,[171] often 4 on one side and 5 on the other with a node on each side in the upper 3 interspaces and others occupying lower interspaces irregularly down to the 6th interspace. Overall 40 of 92 patients (43%) who showed any lymph drainage on LS included internal mammary drainage. Haagensen in his series of patients with breast cancer showed metastases in the internal mammary node field in 28.7% of inner quadrant lesions, 43% of central lesions and 17.1% of outer quadrant cancers (Figure 10.4).[66] Handley's figures for these three regions were 31%, 47% and 16%,[161] percentages which are remarkably consistent with Haagensen's findings. Thus metastases to the internal mammary chain are an important and frequent finding in patients with breast cancer in all quadrants of the breast.

The lymphatic channels which reach the internal mammary chain pass through the posterior surface of the breast, penetrate the pectoralis major muscle and the fascia and then pass through the intercostal space before coursing medially

A

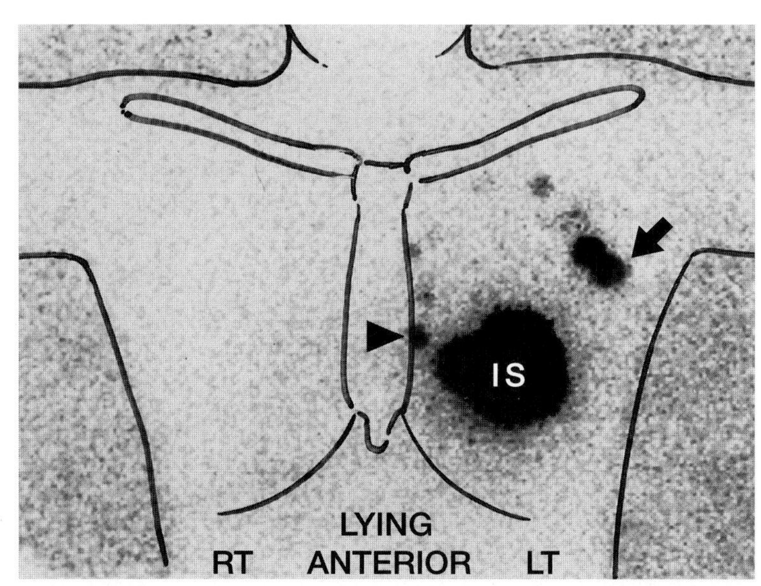

B

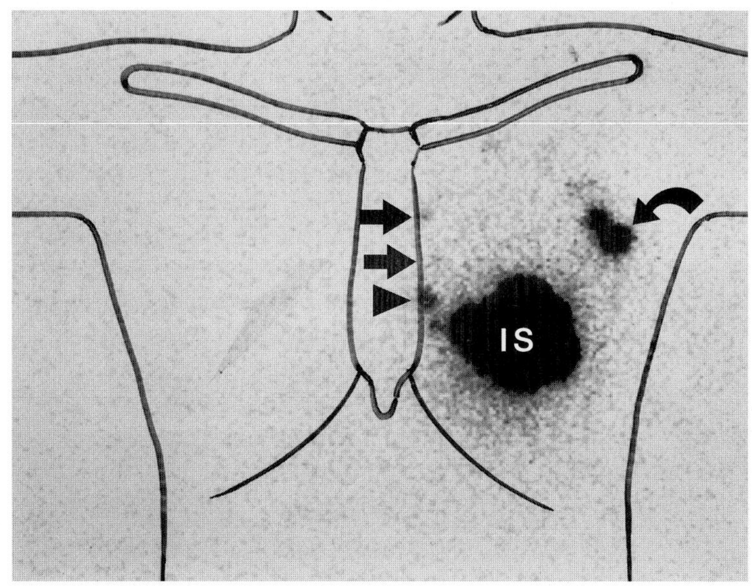

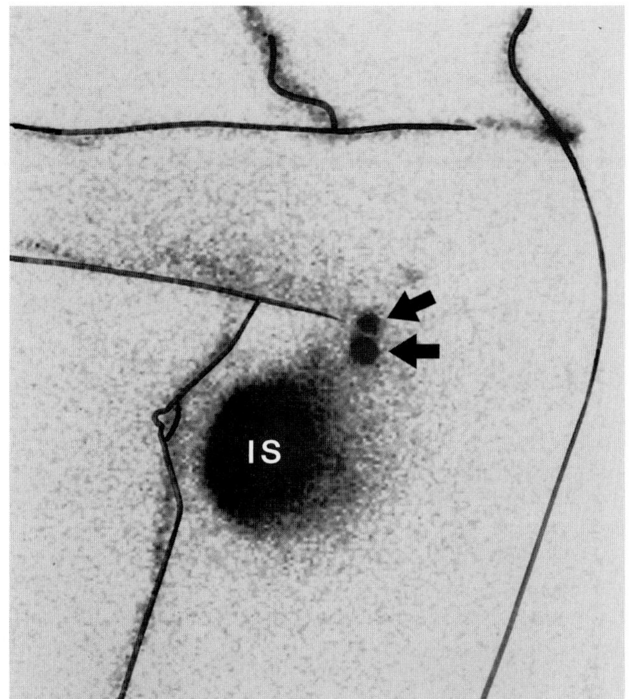

C

Figure 10.3 Lymphoscintigraphy showing internal mammary drainage

A: This dynamic scan in the anterior projection of a patient with a cancer in the left lower inner quadrant close to the nipple shows tracer passing to the left axilla (arrow) and to a node in the left internal mammary chain (arrowhead) at about the level of the third interspace via a curvilinear channel. B: The delayed scan in the anterior projection shows tracer in 2 sentinel nodes in the left axilla (curved arrow) and the sentinel node in the internal mammary chain (arrowhead). There is faint second tier node activity high in the left axilla and two faint nodes higher in the left internal mammary chain (arrows). C: The delayed scan in the left lateral view clearly displays the two left axillary sentinel nodes (arrows).

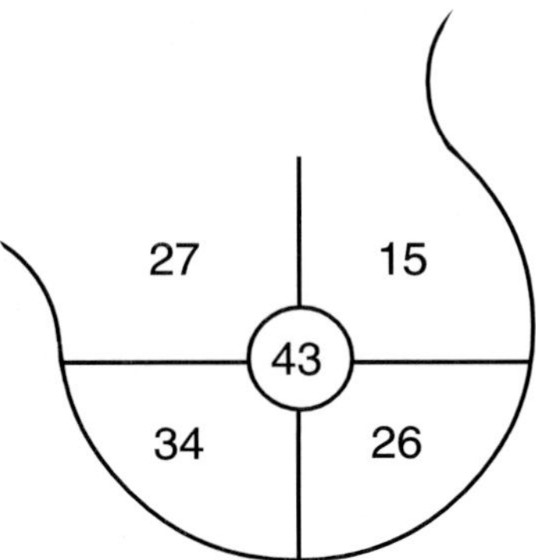

Figure 10.4 The incidence of internal mammary metastases from cancers in the different breast quadrants.

Source: Adapted from Haagensen, C.D., Feind, C.R., Herter, F.P., Slanetz, C.A. and Weinberg, J.A. (1972) *The Lymphatics in Cancer*, p. 583. Philadelphia: W. B. Saunders Co.

to meet the internal mammary lymph nodes. Turner-Warwick found that in some patients the lymph channels coursed laterally to posterior intercostal lymph nodes.[133] This was said to occur when lymph channels perforated the intercostal spaces laterally and below the 6th interspace. We have not yet observed such drainage in our patients.

10.4 SUPRACLAVICULAR DRAINAGE

In the 70 patients with upper quadrant lesions who showed lymph drainage 11 (16%) included direct drainage to the supraclavicular nodes. One patient with a cancer low in the left lower inner quadrant had drainage to the left supraclavicular fossa via an interpectoral node which lay deep to the upper medial aspect of the left breast. The channel appeared to pass on from the interpectoral node to the clavicular node and thus the interpectoral node was the sentinel node and the clavicular node a second tier node (Figure 10.5). This patient had no drainage at all to the axilla or internal mammary nodes. Thus in our 92 patients who showed lymph drainage from the primary cancer site in the breast 11 (12%) showed direct drainage to supraclavicular nodes and one drained exclusively to this area via an interpectoral node.

Past studies which looked at the incidence of metastases in supraclavicular nodes have suggested that these occur generally in conjunction with metastases in the axillary nodes. Haagensen and colleagues[66] felt that metastatic involvement of the supraclavicular nodes occurred usually in a retrograde fashion from involved nodes close to the thoracic duct, in other words only in advanced carcinoma of the breast when the axilla was grossly involved. They did not believe that metastases could occur in the supraclavicular nodes alone. In one large study where supraclavicular nodes were dissected routinely there was an incidence of metastases to this node field in 18% of patients.[174] They also found, however, that there were no metastases in supraclavicular lymph nodes in 149 patients who had no axillary metastases. This latter finding is unexpected in view of the known lymphatic drainage of the breast which we have demonstrated, with 16% of upper quadrant lesions draining directly to the supraclavicular nodes and 12% of lesions overall including supraclavicular drainage. Cruikshank, in his original description of the lymphatic drainage of the breast in 1786, seemed to describe direct drainage from the breast tissue to nodes behind the middle of the clavicle.[52] At the beginning of this century, Mornard demonstrated direct lymphatic drainage from the breast to the supraclavicular nodes in 3% of the subjects he studied, thus the demonstration of direct lymphatic drainage from breast tissue to supraclavicular nodes is not a new finding.[175] With 16% of upper quadrant breast cancers having lymphatic drainage which includes the supraclavicular nodes one would expect metastatic involvement of the supraclavicular nodes in about 40% of these patients, i.e. 6.4% of such patients or 5% or patients with breast cancer generally. It is possible that the microscopic examination of the supraclavicular nodes in these older series missed some true positive cases.

10.5 INTRAMAMMARY INTERVAL NODES

Drainage can sometimes be seen to intramammary interval nodes, which by definition are also sentinel nodes. These can occur anywhere within the breast tissue (Figure 8.1). There were intramammary interval nodes detected in 9 of our 92 patients (10%) who showed lymph flow.

10.6 INTERPECTORAL NODES

It is interesting that in this series we only detected drainage to an interpectoral node in one patient (see Figure 10.5) even though it has been known for some time that these nodes can contain metastases from breast cancer. These nodes, which lie between the pectoralis major and pectoralis minor muscles over the anterior chest wall deep to the mammary gland, were first described by Grossman[172] and soon after by Rotter[127], both of whom stated that metastases occur in these nodes in up to a third of patients. Rotter claimed that metastasis to these nodes could occur early in the disease. It may be that we have sometimes interpreted interpectoral nodes as intramammary interval nodes, but it seems

A

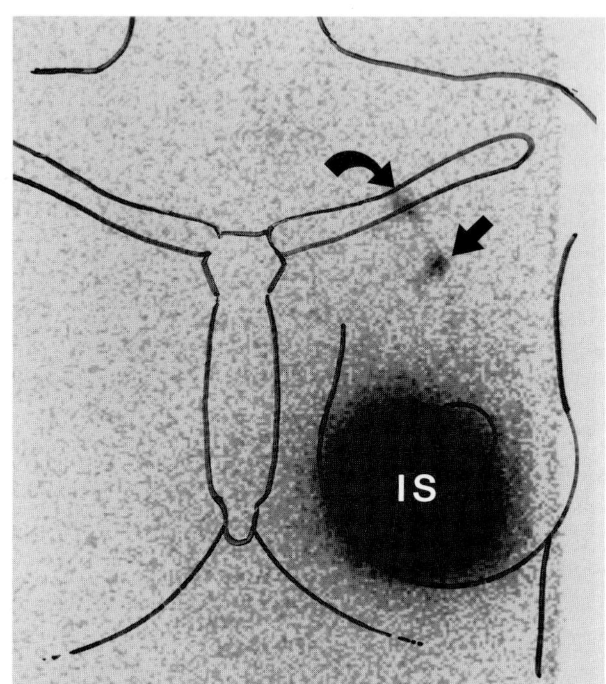

B

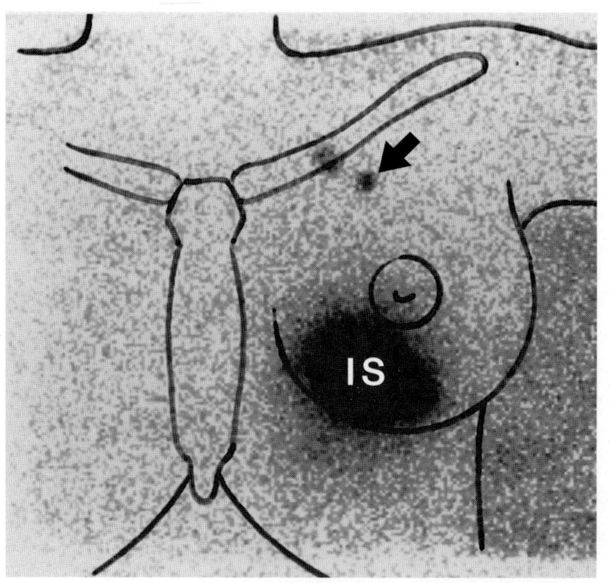

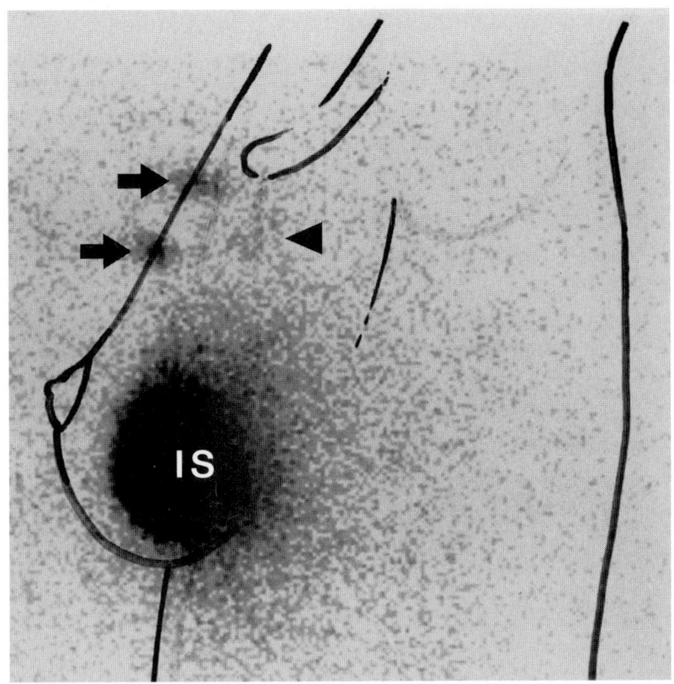

Figure 10.5 Drainage to the supraclavicular fossa via an interpectoral node from a lower quadrant cancer

A: Dynamic lymphoscintigraphy in the anterior projection in a patient with a left lower inner quadrant cancer (IS). In the sitting position a single channel is seen passing upwards to an interpectoral node (arrow) and the breast falls away from the clavicle. The channel appears to continue on to a node in the supraclavicular fossa (curved arrow). B: Delayed scan anteriorly in the supine position shows that the breast lies more superiorly on the chest so that the interpectoral node (arrow) and the supraclavicular node now appear closer together. This illustrates how much the breast can move when the position of imaging is altered and emphasises that the surface location of any node must be marked on the skin in the exact position to be used at surgery. C: In the lateral position a point source is placed on the skin over the location of the interpectoral node and the clavicular node (arrows). Attenuation through breast tissue has made it more difficult to discern but the activity in the interpectoral node (arrowhead) can be seen lying 4 cm deep to the skin.

more likely that activity in these nodes has been obscured by the bloom of activity in the injection sites around the primary tumour. In the patient who showed drainage to an interpectoral node the cancer was in the left lower inner quadrant, well away from the node, and we were therefore able to clearly visualise the node and accurately measure its depth from the skin in the lateral view. The node was 4 cm deep to the skin and at surgery there were 3 cms of soft tissue between the skin mark and the pectoral muscles at this site. The node was thus 1 cm deep to the surface of the pectoral muscles. Though a slight increase in probe counts was found in the area, the surgeon was unable to locate the actual node. The location of these nodes just deep to the mammary gland can make them difficult to discern as separate from the injection site in lateral views. Also, because many of the primary tumours are in the upper outer quadrant of the breast, activity injected around such tumours would directly overlie the interpectoral nodes in the anterior view, thus rendering their detection on scan near impossible. It is also possible that our technique of lymphatic mapping in breast cancer makes it less likely that we will detect lymphatic drainage to the interpectoral nodes. All of our patients received four intramammary injections at the depth of the centre of the tumour in the 12, 3, 6 and 9 o'clock positions. We did not inject deep to the tumour and it is possible that drainage to the interpectoral nodes, when present, occurs from the deep aspect of the tumour. Our injections around the tumour at the depth of its midpoint may thus not detect deep drainage through the back of the breast to interpectoral nodes in all patients who in fact have such drainage.

Since completing this series we have seen a further 2 patients with drainage to interpectoral nodes.

10.7 DRAINAGE ACROSS THE CENTRE LINE OF THE BREAST

Fourteen of 18 inner quadrant lesions (78%) drained to the axilla (4 exclusively) and 17 of 49 outer quadrant lesions (35%) drained to internal mammary nodes (1 exclusively). In all, 46% of lesions drained across the centre line of the breast.

10.8 DRAINAGE FROM LOWER QUADRANTS TO SUPRACLAVICULAR NODES

Drainage from lower quadrants to supraclavicular nodes was only observed in the one patient mentioned earlier (see Figure 10.5). This drainage occurred via an interpectoral node which was the sentinel node in this situation, and we have thus not seen a sentinel node in the supraclavicular region in any patient with a cancer wholely lying in a lower quadrant of the breast.

10.9 DRAINAGE TO OTHER THAN AXILLARY NODES

In 47 of 92 patients (51%) drainage occurred to internal mammary nodes, supraclavicular nodes, an interpectoral node or intramammary interval nodes as well as, or instead of, draining to the axilla. Thus, in 1 of every 2 patients a sentinel node biopsy of the axilla only may have underestimated the extent of lymph node involvement by metastatic disease.

10.10 DRAINAGE DIRECT TO LIVER VIA THE RECTUS ABDOMINIS MUSCLE

Handley described direct spread of breast cancer from the infero-medial aspect of the breast via lymphatics which accompany the superior epigastric blood vessels.[126] These pass down towards the epigastrium, then pass posteriorly through the rectus fascia into the rectus abdominis muscle. The lymphatics then travel upwards to the prepericardial lymph nodes which lie on the upper surface of the diaphragm. These nodes receive other channels from the diaphragm, the falciform ligament and the antero-superior parts of the liver. The prepericardial lymph nodes also form the beginning of the internal mammary chain.

In patients with advanced breast cancer in whom the internal mammary node chain is blocked by metastatic disease, this lymphatic route can allow the retrograde spread of cancer cells from the lower medial part of the breast directly to the liver.

We have not yet seen any breast cancer patient display this drainage pattern via the epigastrium to prepericardial nodes. None of our patients had advanced disease and with the modern emphasis on early diagnosis of breast cancer it is unlikely that this drainage pathway will be demonstrated on lymphatic mapping studies today.

10.11 DRAINAGE TO THE CONTRALATERAL BREAST AND AXILLA

It would seem that in normal adults lymphatic drainage from the breast does not occur to the contralateral breast or to contralateral node fields in the axilla, supraclavicular and internal mammary chains.[133] We did not demonstrate direct contralateral drainage in any of our patients, however we have seen tracer pass onward from sentinel nodes in the ipsilateral internal mammary chain to second tier nodes in the contralateral internal mammary chain. Following surgery however this would appear to occur in some patients. We have shown drainage using lymphoscintigraphy from the skin of the right arm to the left axilla in a patient who had previously undergone a right axillary node clearance for melanoma. Others have shown similar findings using lymphangiography, though the cases described by Bobbio and colleagues were also from the right side to the left axilla and they did not observe such drainage from left to right.[173] It would also seem possible that such contralateral drainage could occur in patients with very advanced disease due to completely blocked lymphatic drainage pathways on the side of the cancer.

10.12 THE CONCEPT OF 'SKIP' METASTASES

For some time surgeons have debated the occurrence and importance of so-called 'skip' metastases. This describes the situation in which axillary Level I or Level II lymph nodes are tumour free and metastases are found in Level II or III respectively, or in supraclavicular nodes. These were thought to be caused by tumour cells passing through a lymph node onwards to a higher level node, thus "skipping" the first node. The results of lymphoscintigraphy, however, make it almost certain that this phenomenon simply represents direct lymphatic drainage to a higher level node without passage through the filter function of any lower level lymph nodes.

10.13 SECOND TIER LYMPH NODES IN BREAST CANCER

As in cutaneous lymphoscintigraphy, the best way to distinguish second tier nodes from sentinel nodes is to identify the lymphatic vessel entering the sentinel node and passing onwards to the second tier node when present. Second tier nodes are often seen in the axilla and the internal mammary chain. If no dominant channel is seen on early imaging they can generally be identified as they lie more centrally in the node field and have much less activity than the sentinel node or nodes. Second tier nodes can be seen using any radiocolloid and are not just seen when smaller particle colloids are used for lymphatic mapping. Remember, not all 'hot' nodes are sentinel nodes. In a recent report, Gulec and colleagues using filtered 99mTc sulphur colloid reported in a series of 32 patients with breast cancer, 1 patient with 6 sentinel nodes in the axilla, 2 with 5, 2 with 4, and 7 with 3 sentinel nodes in the axilla.[176] These sentinel nodes had been identified as 'hot' with a gamma probe at surgery. Lymphoscintigraphy was not performed to identify the sentinel nodes. In our patients using lymphoscintigraphy and 99mTc antimony sulphide colloid which has a smaller particle size than Gulec's radiocolloid, we have seen 81 patients with 1 sentinel nodes in the axilla, 6 with 2, and only 1 with more than 2 sentinel nodes in the axilla. This patient had 4 sentinel nodes. The clear implication of this data is that Gulec and colleagues are removing radioactive non-sentinel second and possibly third tier lymph nodes. This is not the intent of the sentinel lymph node biopsy procedure. We believe it is not possible to perform accurate sentinel lymph node biopsy using radioactive tracers without high quality lymphoscintigraphy using appropriately sized radiocolloids.

Chapter 11

THE FUTURE

11.1 LYMPHOSCINTIGRAPHY

Until now lymphatic mapping techniques have concentrated on accurately mapping the lymphatic system using appropriately sized colloid particles which gain access to the lumen of the lymphatic capillaries under physiological conditions. This approach also relies on physiological processes in the draining lymph nodes such as opsonisation and phagocytosis to trap and retain the colloid in the node. This still means that the majority of the injected radiocolloid will remain at the injection site. In the future it may be possible to develop radiopharmaceuticals which migrate more effectively and rapidly through the lymphatics to the draining sentinel nodes but which are more completely retained in the node because of strong binding to receptors or increased phagocytosis in the node. Some work in this area has already been reported.[82,83]

Current imaging protocols for lymphoscintigraphy in melanoma and breast cancer patients will need to be modified to ensure that all sentinel nodes are detected. This will mean checking for drainage to the triangular intermuscular space, paravertebral and retroperitoneal nodes and the epitrochlear and popliteal nodes when relevant in melanoma patients. In breast cancer patients with lower outer quadrant tumours a posterior view should be performed to detect drainage to posterior intercostal nodes when present.

11.2 SURGICAL TECHNIQUE

Why perform SLNB on just the axillary node field in breast cancer patients? It is known that the presence of nodal metastases in the axilla of breast cancer patients has an adverse effect on their prognosis. If metastases occur in lymph node basins in proportion to the incidence of lymphatic drainage to that area as shown on lymphoscintigraphy then based on our data just over half the patients will have micrometastases in internal mammary, supraclavicular, interpectoral or intramammary interval lymph nodes.[166] Since it is possible to obtain an accurate map of peritumoral lymphatic drainage in most patients it seems illogical to ignore the sentinel nodes in these areas. Based on our present knowledge of the patterns of lymphatic drainage in breast cancer it is logical to assume that in some patients the non-axillary sentinel nodes will be the only nodes with metastases. For this reason we believe that in the future, sentinel nodes in the supraclavicular and internal mammary lymph node fields, as well as interpectoral nodes when present, will be resected along with any axillary sentinel nodes and intramammary interval nodes. In this way the true nodal status of each patient with breast cancer will be determined.[170] Early attempts at biopsying sentinel nodes outside the axilla have recently been described and some of these sentinel nodes have been positive for metastases.[177] With this knowledge, more precise therapeutic decision making should be possible.

Improvements in the design of gamma detecting probes for intraoperative use are likely. Probes with a better ergonomic design which are easier for the surgeon to manipulate in the surgical field will speed up the location of the radiolabelled sentinel node. Increasing the sensitivity of the probe would also be a useful advance especially when surgery is to be performed the day after lymphoscintigraphy when node counts will have fallen markedly. Improving collimation will also make the probes more accurate in directing surgery towards the radiolabelled node.

11.3 HISTOLOGICAL ASSESSMENT

In both melanoma and breast cancer patients it may be possible to facilitate the accurate histological examination of a sentinel node by concentrating on the part of the node which directly receives tracer. Including a small amount of carbon black with the injected tracer has been suggested. This would enable the area to be seen microscopically and perhaps simplify the procedure. Other refinements to the histological examination of sentinel lymph nodes are also likely to become more widely used, such as assessment using a reverse transcriptase polymerase chain reaction (RT-PCR) assay for tyrosinase messenger RNA, which is found almost exclusively in melanocytes. This can detect the presence of only one or two metastatic cells in a lymph node containing millions of cells. The significance of detecting such tiny amounts of metastatic tumour, however, will need to be determined by further study.[178,179]

11.4 OTHER CANCERS

Patients with other cancers which have lymphatic spread as a feature of their natural history should also benefit from lymphatic mapping and sentinel node biopsy. These include patients with cancers of the penis, vulva, bowel, pancreas, thyroid and lung. Early studies have already been undertaken in several of these tumours and preliminary results appear promising.

Chapter 12

CONCLUSIONS

Experience to date with lymphatic mapping of the skin and breast has highlighted the enormous interpatient variation in the patterns of lymph drainage which occurs and has confirmed that it is not possible to predict the pattern of drainage in an individual patient. The combination of lymphatic mapping and sentinel node biopsy appears likely to revolutionise the practice of surgical oncology in melanoma and breast cancer patients and it is becoming increasingly clear that without lymphatic mapping, rational treatment of regional lymph nodes in these patients is simply not possible. It also seems probable that the use of these techniques in patients with other tumours will prove of benefit.

REFERENCES

1. Ryan, T.J. (1975) The Lymphatics of the Skin. In *The Physiology and Pathophysiology of the Skin*, vol. 3, edited by Jarrett, pp. 1755–1780. London: Academic Press.
2. Sabin, F.R. (1904) On the development of the superficial lymphatics in the skin of the pig. *Am J Anat*, **3**, 183.
3. Ranvier (1895) Developpement des vaisseaux lymphatiques. *C R Academie des Sciences*, 1105.
4. Slavin, S.A., Upton, J., Kaplan, W.D., and van den Abbeele, A.D. (1997) An investigation of lymphatic function following free-tissue transfer. *Plast Reconstr Surg*, **99**, 730–741.
5. Romani, J.D. (1973) Etudes des capillaires lymphatique du derme chez les diabetiques. *Angeiologie*, **25**, 227–236.
6. Fawcett, D.W. (1961) Intercellular bridges. *Expl Cell Res*, **8**, 174.
7. Leak, L.V. (1980) Lymphatic vessels. In *Cardiovascular System, Lymphoreticular and Hematopoietic System*, edited by J.V. Johannessen, pp. 159–183. New York: McGraw-Hill.
8. Gerli, R., Ibba, L. and Fruschelli, C. (1991) Ultrastructural cytochemistry of anchoring filaments of human lymphatic capillaries and their relation to elastic fibres. *Lymphology*, **24**, 105–112.
9. Braverman, I.M. and Yen, A. (1974) Microcirculation in the psoriatic skin. *J Invest Dermatol*, **62**, 493–502.
10. Leak, L.V. (1970) Electron microscopic observations on lymphatic capillaries and the structural components of the connective tissue-lymph interface. *Microvasc Res*, **2**, 361–391.
11. Haagansen, C.D., Feind, C.R., Herter, F.P. et al. (1972) Lymphatics of the trunk. In *The Lymphatics in Cancer*, edited by C.D. Haagansen, pp. 437–458. Philadelphia: W. B. Saunders Co.
12. Berk, D.A., Swartz, M.A., Leu, A.J. and Jain, R.K. (1996) Transport in lymphatic capillaries. II. Microscopic velocity measurement with fluorescence photobleaching. *Am J Physiol*, **270**, H330–H337.
13. Navas, V., O'Morchoe, P.J. and O'Morchoe, C.C. (1991) Lymphatic valves of the rat pancreas. *Lymphology*, **24**, 146–154.

14. Pollard, T.D. and Weihing, R.R. (1974) Actin and myosin and cell movement. *CRC Crit Rev Biochem*, **2**, 1–65.
15. Sappey, M.P.C. (1874) *Anatomie, Physiologie, Pathologie des vaisseaux Lymphatiques consideres chez L'homme at les Vertebres*, edited by A. DeLahaye and E. Lecrosnier. Paris
16. Zhang, J. and Xiu, R. (1995) The characteristics of spontaneous rhythmical microlymphomotion. *Chung Hua I Hsueh Tsa Chih*, **75**, 262–265.
17. Mislin, H. (1976) Active contractility of the lymphangion and co-ordination of lymphangion chains. *Experientia*, **32**, 820–822.
18. Kinmouth, J.B. and Taylor, G.W. (1956) Spontaneous rhythmic contractility in human lymphatics. *J Physiol(Lond)*, **133**, 3.
19. Forkert, P.G., Thliveris, J.A. and Bertalanffy, F.D. (1977) Structure of sinuses in the human lymph node. *Cell Tissue Res*, **183**, 115–130.
20. Gowans, J.L. and Knight, E.T. (1964) Circulation of small lymphocytes. *Proc R Soc London*, **159**, 257.
21. Sainte-Marie, G., Sin, Y.M. and Chan, C. (1967) The diapedesis of lymphocytes through postcapillary venules of rat lymph nodes. *Rev Can Biol*, **26**, 141–151.
22. Nichols, W.S. and Chisari, F.V. (1990) Structure and function of the lymphoid tissues. In *Hematology* (4th edn), edited by W.J. Williams, E. Beutler, A.J. Erslev and M.A. Lichtman, pp. 49–50. New York: McGraw-Hill.
23. Nopajaroonsri, C. and Simon, G.T. (1971) Phagocytosis of colloidal carbon in a lymph node. *Am J Pathol*, **65**, 25–42.
24. Ludwig, J. (1962) Ueber kurschlusswege der lymphbahnen und ihre beziehungen zur lymphogen krebsmetastasierung. *Path Microbiol*, **25**, 329.
25. Auche, J. (1930) De la neo-formation des ganglions lymphatiques. *Rev Chir*, **68**, 350.
26. Shields, J.W. (1992) Lymph, lymph glands, and homeostasis. *Lymphology*, **25**, 147–153.
27. Pappenheimer, J.R., Renkin, E.M. and Borrero, L.M. (1951) Filtration, diffusion and molecular sieving through peripheral capillary membranes. A contribution to the pore theory of capillary permeability. *Am J Physiol*, **167**, 13.
28. Leak, L.V. (1971) Studies on the permeability of lymphatic capillaries. *J Cell Biol*, **50**, 300–323.
29. Allen, L. (1938) Volume and pressure changes in terminal lymphatics. *Am J Physiol*, **123**, 3–4.
30. Franzeck, U.K., Fischer, M., Costanzo, U., Herrig, I. and Bollinger, A. (1996) Effect of postural changes on human lymphatic capillary pressure of the skin. *J Physiol*, **494**, 595–600.
31. Spiegel, M., Vesti, B., Shore, A. et al. (1992) Pressure of lymphatic capillaries in human skin. *Am J Physiol*, **262**, H1208–H1210.

32. Delamere, G., Poirier, P. and Cuneo, B. (1903) The Lymphatics. In *A Treatise of Human Anatomy*, edited by P.P. Charpy. Westminster: Archibald Constable and Co. Ltd.
33. Yoffey, J.M. and Courtice, F.C. (1970) *Lymphatics, Lymph and the Lymphomyeloid Complex*. London: Academic Press.
34. Gangon, W.F. (ed) (1979) *Review of Medical Physiology*. Los Altos: Lange Medical Publications.
35. Gulec, S.A., Moffat, F.L. and Carroll, R.G. (1997) The expanding clinical role for intraoperative gamma probes. In *Nuclear Medicine Annual 1997*, edited by L.M. Freeman. Philadelphia: Lippincott-Raven.
36. Jacobsson, S. and Kjellmer, L. (1964) Flow and protein content of lymph in resting and exercising skeletal muscle. *Acta Physiol Scand*, **60**, 278–285.
37. Crandell, L.A., Barker, S.B. and Graham, D.G. (1943) A study of the lymph flow from a patient with thoracic duct fistula. *Gastroenterology*, **1**, 1040–1048.
38. Langer, K., Seidler, C. and Partsch, H. (1996) Ultrastructural study of the dermal microvasculature in patients undergoing retrograde intravenous pressure infusions. *Dermatology*, **192**, 103–109.
39. Fischer, M., Franzeck, U.K., Herrig, I. et al. (1996) Flow velocity of single lymphatic capillaries in human skin. *Am J Physiol*, **270**, H358–H363.
40. Swartz, M.A., Berk, D.A. and Jain, R.K. (1996) Transport in lymphatic capillaries. I. Macroscopic measurements using residence time distribution theory. *Am J Physiol*, **270**, H324–H329.
41. Uren, R.F., Howman-Giles, R.B., Thompson, J.F., Roberts, J. and Bernard, E. (1998) Variability of cutaneous lymphatic flow rates. *Melanoma Res.*, **8**, 279.
42. Casley-Smith, J.R. (1977) *Lymph and Lymphatics in Microcirculation*, edited by G. Kaley and B.M. Altura, pp. 423–502. University Park Press.
43. McMaster, P.D. (1937) Changes in the cutaneous lymphatics of human beings and in the lymph flow under normal and pathologic conditions. *J Exp Med*, **65**, 347–372.
44. White, J.C., Field, M.E. and Drinker, C.K. (1933) On the protein content and normal flow of lymph from the foot of the dog. *Am J Physiol*, **103**, 34–44.
45. McHale, N.G. and Roddie, I.C. (1976) The effect of transmural pressure on pumping activity in isolated bovine lymphatic vessels. *J Physiol*, **261**, 255–269.
46. Drake, R.E., Dhother, S., Oppenlander, V.M. and Gabel, J.C. (1996) Lymphatic pump function curves in awake sheep. *Am J Physiol*, **270**, R486–R488.
47. Sjoberg, T. and Steen, S. (1991) Contractile properties of lymphatics from the human lower leg. *Lymphology*, **24**, 16–21.
48. Mortimer, P.S. (1995) Evaluation of lymphatic function: abnormal lymph drainage in venous disease. *Int Angiol*, **14**, 32–35.

49. Massa, N. (1532) *Lib Introd Anat.*
50. Aselli, G. (1627) *De Lactibus sive Lacteis Venis.* Milan: J B Bidellius.
51. Pecquet, J. (1653) *New Anatomical Experiments* (English translation). London: O Pulleyn.
52. Cruikshank (1786) *The Anatomy of the Absorbing Vessels of the Human Body.*
53. Hewson (1771) Experimental inquiries on the blood, with some remarks on it and an appendix relating to the lymphatic system in birds, fishes and amphibious animals. London.
54. Mascagni (1787) *Vasorum Lymphaticorum Corporis Humani Historia et Ichnographia.* Sienne: P Carli.
55. Lauth (1824) *Essai sur les Vaisseaux Lymphatiques.* Strasbourg.
56. Recklinghausen, FDv (1862) *Die Lymphgefasse und ihre Beziehung zum Bindegewebe.* Berlin: A. Hirschwald.
57. Regaud (1894) Origine des vaisseaux lymphatiques de la mamelle. *C R Soc Biol*, **20**, 495.
58. Ranvier (1894) Chyliferes du rat. *C R Acad Sciences*, **12**, 621.
59. Kytmanoff (1901) Ueber die nervenendigungen in den lymphgefassen der saugethiere. *Anat Anzeig*, **15**.
60. Gerota (1896) Zur technik der lymphgefassinjection. Eine neue injectionsmasse fur lymphgefasse. Polychrom. Injection. *Anat Anzeiger*, **12**, 216.
61. Bartels, P. (1909) Das lymphgefasssystem. In *Handbuch der Anatomie des Menschen* (4th part), edited by Kv. Bardeleben. Jena: Gustav Fischer.
62. Gray, J.H. (1939) The relation of lymphatic vessels to the spread of cancer. *Br J Surg*, **26**, 462.
63. Horta, J.D., DaMotta, L.C., Abbatt, J.D. and Roriz, M.L. (1965) Malignancy and other late effects following administration of Thorotrast. *Lancet*, **2**, 201.
64. Hudack, S. and McMaster, P.D. (1933) The lymphatic participation in human cutaneous phenomena. *J Exp Med*, **57**, 751.
65. Strug, L.H., Leon, W. and Cohn, I.J. (1954) Vital staining of lymphatics during surgery, *Surg Forum Am Coll Surg.* Philadelphia: W. B. Saunders Co.
66. Haagensen, C.D., Feind, C.R., Herter, F.P., Slanetz, C.A. and Weinberg, J.A. (1972) *The Lymphatics in Cancer*, p. 583. Philadelphia: W. B. Saunders Co.
67. Kinmonth, J. (1952) Lymphangiography in man; a method of outlining lymphatic trunks at operation. *Clin Sci*, **11**, 13–20.
68. Clouse, M.E. and Wallace, S. (eds) (1985) Lymphatic Imaging. In *Lymphography, Computed Tomography and Scintigraphy* (2nd edn), pp. 15–21. Baltimore: Williams and Wilkins.
69. Sherman, A. and Ter-Pogossian, M. (1953) Lymph node concentration of radioactive colloidal gold following interstitial injection. *Cancer*, **6**, 1238–1240.

70. Aspegren, K., Strand, S.E. and Persson, B.R. (1978) Quantitative lymphoscintigraphy for detection of metastases to the internal mammary lymph nodes. Biokinetics of 99mTc-sulphur colloid uptake and correlation with microscopy. *Acta Radiol Oncol*, **17**, 17–26.
71. Kaplan, W.D., Davis, M.A. and Rose, C.M. (1979) A comparison of two technetium-99m-labeled radiopharmaceuticals for lymphoscintigraphy. *J Nucl Med*, **20**, 933–937.
72. Ege, G.N. and Warbick, A. (1979) Lymphoscintigraphy: a comparison of 99Tc(m)-antimony sulphide colloid and 99Tc(m)-stannous phytate. *Br J Radiol*, **52**, 124–129.
73. Strand, S.E. and Persson, B.R. (1979) Quantitative lymphoscintigraphy I: basic concepts for optimal uptake of radiocolloids in the parasternal lymph nodes of rabbits. *J Nucl Med*, **20**, 1038–1046.
74. Nagai, K., Ito, Y., Otsuka, N. et al. (1981) Experimental studies on uptake of 99mTc-antimony sulfide colloid in RES. A comparison with various 99mTc-colloids. *Int J Nucl Med Biol*, **8**, 85–89.
75. Nathanson, S.D., Nelson, L. & Karvelis, K.C. (1996) Rates of flow of technetium 99m-labeled human serum albumin from peripheral injection sites to sentinel lymph nodes. *Ann Surg Oncol*, **3**, 329–335.
76. Uren, R.F., Howman-Giles, R.B. and Thompson, J.F. (1997) Variation in cutaneous lymphatic flow rates. *Ann Surg Oncol*, **4**, 279–280.
77. Albertini, J.J., Lyman, G.H., Cox, C., et al. (1996) Lymphatic mapping and sentinel node biopsy in the patient with breast cancer. *JAMA*, **276**, 1818–1822.
78. Schmidt, M.S., Gardner, P.M., Redlich, P.N., et al. (1998) Breast lymphoscintigraphy: High-volume injection technique improves sentinel lymph node visualization. *J Nucl Med*, **39**, 25P.
79. Eary, J.F., Mankoff, D.A., Dunnwald, L.K., et al. (1998) Sentinel node lymphatic mapping for breast cancer: Application to a diverse patient population. *J Nucl Med*, **39**, 24P.
80. Bergqvist, L., Strand, S-E. and Persson, B.R. (1983) Particle sizing and biokinetics of interstitial lymphoscintigraphic agents. *Semin Nucl Med*, **8**, 9–19.
81. Frier, M. (1981) Phagocytosis. In *Progress in Radiopharmacology*, edited by P.M. Cox, pp. 249–260. Amsterdam: Elsevier/North Holland Biomedical Press.
82. Moghimi, S.M., Hawley, A.E., Christy, N.M. et al. (1994) Surface engineered nanospheres with enhanced drainage into lymphatics and uptake by macrophages of the regional lymph nodes. *FEBS Lett*, **344**, 25–30.
83. Vera, D.R., Wisner, E.R. and Stadalnik, R.C. (1997) Sentinel node imaging via a nonparticulate receptor-binding radiotracer. *J Nucl Med*, **38**, 530–535.

84. Kapteijn, B.A., Nieweg, O.E., Muller, S.H., et al. (1997) Validation of gamma probe detection of the sentinel node in melanoma. *J Nucl Med*, **38**, 362–366.
85. Thompson, J.F., Niewind, P., Uren, R.F. et al. (1997) Single-dose isotope injection for both preoperative lymphoscintigraphy and intraoperative sentinel lymph node identification in melanoma patients. *Melanoma Res*, **7**, 500–506.
86. Uren, R.F., Howman-Giles, R.B. and Thompson, J.F. (1998) Demonstration of second tier lymph nodes during preoperative lymphoscintigraphy for melanoma: Incidence varies with primary tumour site. *Ann Surg Oncol*, **5**, 517–521
87. Walker, L. (1950) Localization of radioactive colloids in lymph nodes. *J Lab Clin Med*, **36**, 440–449.
88. Nathanson, S.D., Anaya, P., Karvelis, K.C., Eck, L. and Havstad, S. (1997) Sentinel lymph node uptake of two different technetium-labeled radiocolloids. *Ann Surg Oncol*, **4**, 104–110.
89. Dornfest, B.S., Lenehan, P.F., Reilly, T.M. et al. (1977) Effects of sera of normal, anemic and leukemic rats on particle size distribution of 99mtTchnetium-sulfur colloid in vitro. *J Reticuloendothel Soc*, **21**, 317–329.
90. Alazraki, N.P., Eshima, D., Eshima, L.A. et al. (1997) Lymphoscintigraphy, the sentinel node concept, and the intraoperative gamma probe in melanoma, breast cancer, and other potential cancers. *Semin Nucl Med*, **27**, 55–67.
91. Wong, J.H., Terada, K., Ko, P. and Coel, M.N. (1998) Lack of effect of particle size on the identification of the sentinel node in cutaneous malignancies. *Ann Surg Oncol*, **5**, 77–80.
92. Tonakie, A., Yahanda, A., Sondak, V. and Wahl, R.L. (1998) Reproducibility of lymphoscintigraphic drainage patterns in sequential TC-99M HSA and TC-99M sulfur colloid studies: implications for sentinel node identification in melanoma. *J Nucl Med*, **39**, 25P.
93. Glass, E.C., Essner, R. and Morton, D.L. (in press) Kinetics of three lymphoscintigraphic agents in patients with cutaneous melanoma. *J Nucl Med.*
94. Bronskill, M.J. (1983) Radiation dose estimates for interstitial radiocolloid lymphoscintigraphy. *Semin Nucl Med*, **13**, 20–25.
95. Uren, R., Commens, C. and Howman-Giles, R. (1994) Intradermal injections - a potential health hazard? *Med J Aust*, **161**, 226.
96. Uren, R.F., Howman-Giles, R., Thompson, J.F. et al. (1996) Lymphatic drainage to triangular intermuscular space lymph nodes in melanoma on the back. *J Nucl Med*, **37**, 964–966.
97. Uren, R.F., Howman-Giles, R.B., Shaw, H.M., Thompson, J.F. and McCarthy, W.H. (1993) Lymphoscintigraphy in high-risk melanoma of the

trunk: predicting draining node groups, defining lymphatic channels and locating the sentinel node. *J Nucl Med*, **34**, 1435–1440.

98. Uren, R.F., Howman-Giles, R.B. and Thompson, J.F. (1998) Lymphatic drainage from the skin of the back to intra-abdominal lymph nodes in melanoma patients. *Ann Surg Oncol*, **5**, 384–387.
99. Uren, RF, Howman-Giles, R.B., Thompson, J.F., Shaw, H.M. and McCarthy, W.H. (1995) Lymphatic drainage from peri-umbilical skin to internal mammary nodes. *Clin Nucl Med*, **20**, 254–255.
100. Uren, RF, Howman-Giles, R., Thompson, J.F., Quinn, M.J. (1996) Direct lymphatic drainage from the skin of the forearm to a supraclavicular node. *Clin Nucl Med*, **21**, 387–389.
101. Uren, R.F., Roberts, J., Howman-Giles, R.B. and Thompson, J.F. (1996) Direct lymphatic drainage from the skin of the elbow to an interpectoral node. *Regional Cancer Treatment*, **9**, 100–102.
102. O'Brien, C.J., Uren, R.F., Thompson, J.F. et al. (1995) Prediction of potential metastatic sites in cutaneous head and neck melanoma using lymphoscintigraphy. *Am J Surg*, **170**, 461–466.
103. Uren, R.F., Howman-Giles, R., Thompson, J.F., et al. (1994) Lymphoscintigraphy to identify sentinel nodes in patients with melanoma. *Melanoma Res*, **4**, 395–399.
104. Morton, D.L., Wen, D-R., Wong, J.H. et al. (1992) Technical details of intraoperative lymphatic mapping for early stage melanoma. *Arch Surg*, **127**, 392–399.
105. Cabanas, R.M. (1977) An approach for the treatment of penile carcinoma. *Cancer*, **39**, 456–466.
106. Bouchot, O., Bouvier, S., Bochereau, G. and Jeddi, M. (1993) Cancer of the penis: the value of systematic biopsy of the superficial inguinal lymph nodes in clinical N0 stage patients. *Prog Urol*, **3**, 228–233.
107. Pettaway, C.A., Pisters, L.L., Dinney, C.P. et al. (1995) Sentinel lymph node dissection for penile carcinoma: the M. D. Anderson Cancer Center experience. *J Urol*, **154**, 1999–2003.
108. Krag, D.N., Meijer, S.J., Weaver, D.L. et al. (1995) Minimal-access surgery for staging of malignant melanoma. *Arch Surg*, **130**, 654–658.
109. Pijpers, R., Borgstein, P.J., Meijer, S. et al. (1997) Sentinel node biopsy in melanoma patients: dynamic lymphoscintigraphy followed by intraoperative gamma probe and vital dye guidance. *World J Surg*, **21**, 788–793.
110. McCarthy, W.H., Thompson, J.F. and Uren, R.F. (1995) Invited Commentary on "Minimal-access surgery for staging of malignant melanoma" by Krag et al. *Arch Surg*, **130**, 659–660.
111. Sugarbaker, E.V. and McBride, C.M. (1976) Melanoma of the trunk: the results of surgical excision and anatomic guidelines for predicting nodal metastasis. *Surgery*, **80**, 22–30.

112. Fee, H.J., Robinson, D.S., Sample, W.F. et al. (1978) The determination of lymph shed by colloidal gold scanning in patients with malignant melanoma: a preliminary study. *Surgery*, **84**, 626–632.
113. Meyer, C.M., Lecklitner, M.L., Logic, J.R. et al. (1979) Technetium-99m sulfur-colloid cutaneous lymphoscintigraphy in the management of truncal melanoma. *Radiology*, **131**, 205–209.
114. Sullivan, D.C., Croker, B.P., Harris, C.C., Deery, P. and Seigler, H.F. (1981) Lymphoscintigraphy in malignant melanoma: 99m-Tc antimony sulfur colloid. *Am J Roentgenol*, **137**, 847–851.
115. Bergqvist, L., Strand, S.E., Hafstrom, L. and Jonsson, P.E. (1984) Lymphoscintigraphy in patients with malignant melanoma: a quantitative and qualitative evaluation of its usefulness. *Eur J Nucl Med*, **9**, 129–135.
116. Norman, J., Cruse, C.W., Espinosa, C. et al. (1991) Redefinition of cutaneous lymphatic drainage with the use of lymphoscintigraphy for malignant melanoma. *Am J Surg*, **162**, 432–437.
117. Eberbach, M.A. and Wahl, R.L. (1989) Lymphatic anatomy: functional nodal basins. *Ann Plast Surg*, **22**, 25–31.
118. Uren, R.F., Howman-Giles, R.B., Thompson, J.F. and McCarthy, W.H. (1998) Exclusive lymphatic drainage from a melanoma on the back to intra-abdominal lymph nodes. *Clin Nucl Med*, **23**, 71–73.
119. Robbins, K.T., Medina, J.E., Wolfe, G.T. et al. (1991) Standardizing neck dissection terminology. Official report of the Academy's committee for head and neck surgery and oncology. *Arch Otolaryngol Head Neck Surg*, **117**, 601–605.
120. O'Brien,C.J., Petersen-Schaefer, K., Ruark, D. et al. (1995) Radical, modified, and selective neck dissection for cutaneous malignant melanoma. *Head Neck*, **17**, 232–241.
121. Rouviere, H. (1938) Anatomy of the human lymphatic system. Ann Arbor, MI: Edwards Brothers.
122. Hunt, J.A., Thompson, J.F., Uren, R.F., Howman-Giles, R.B. and Harman, C.R. (1998) Epitrochlear lymph nodes as a site of melanoma metastasis. *Ann of Surg*, **5**, 248–252.
123. Kinmouth, J.B., Taylor, G.W. and Harper, R.K. (1955) Lymphography: a technique for its clinical use in the lower limb. *Br Med J*, **1**, 940.
124. Browse, N.L. (1972) Normal lymphographic appearances of the lower limb and axilla. In *The Lymphatics: Diseases, Lymphography and Surgery*, edited by J.B. Kinmouth. Baltimore: Williams and Wilkins.
125. Hunt, J.A., Thompson, J.F., Uren, R.F., Howman-Giles, R.B., Harman, C.R. (in press) Popliteal lymph node involvement by metastatic melanoma. *Melanoma Res*.
126. Handley, W.S. (1927) Parasternal invasion of thorax in breast cancer and its suppression by use of radium tubes as operative precaution. *Surg Gynecol Obstet*, **45**, 721.

127. Rotter, J. (1899) Zur topographie des mammacarcinoms. *Arch f klin Chir*, **58**, 346.
128. Halsell, J.T. et al. (1965) Lymphatic drainage of the breast demonstrated by vital dye staining and radiography. *Ann Surg*, **162**, 221.
129. Kendall, B.E., Arthur, J.F., Patey, D.H. (1963) Lymphangiography in carcinoma of the breast. *Cancer*, **16**, 1233.
130. Desprez-Curely, J.P., Bismuth, V., Fron, P. and Bourdon, R. (1963) La lymphographie du membre superieur dans les affections tumorales malignes. *Ann Radiol*, **6**, 437.
131. Pickren, J.W. (1956) Lymphnode metastasis in carcinoma of the female mammary gland. *Bull Roswell Park Memorial Inst*, **1**, 79.
132. Hultborn, K.A., Larsson, L.G. and Ragnhult, I. (1955) The lymph drainage from the breast to the axillary and parasternal lymph nodes, studied with the aid of colloidal AU198. *Acta Radiol*, **43**, 52.
133. Turner-Warwick, R.T. (1959) The lymphatics of the breast. *Br J Surg*, **46**, 574.
134. Vendrell-Torne, E., Setpoain-Quinquer, J., Domenech-Torne, F.M. (1972) Study of normal mammary lymphatic drainage using radioactive isotopes. *J Nucl Med*, **13**, 801–805.
135. McLean, R.G. and Ege, G.N. (1986) Prognostic value of axillary lymphoscintigraphy in breast carcinoma patients. *J Nucl Med*, **27**, 1116–1124.
136. Gitsch, E., Philipp, K. and Kubista, E. (1983) Intraoperative lymphoscintigraphy in radical surgery of cancer. *Geburtshilfe Frauenheilkd*, **43**, 112–115.
137. Bourgeois, P., Fruhling, J. and Henry, J. (1983) Postoperative axillary lymphoscintigraphy in the management of breast cancer. *Int J Radiat Oncol Biol Phys*, **9**, 29–32.
138. Gabelle, P., Comet, M., Bodin, J.P. et al. (1981) Mammary lymphatic scintiscans by intratumoral injection in the assessment of breast cancer. *Nouv Presse Med*, **10**, 3067–3070.
139. Serin, D., Vinot, J.M., Martin, P. et al. (1986) The value of breast lymphoscintigraphy in the definition of axillary staging in cancer of the breast. *Bull Cancer* (Paris), **73**, 299–304.
140. Gasparini, M., Andreoli, C., Rodari, A., Costa, A. and Buraggi, G.L. (1987) Lack of efficacy of lymphoscintigraphy in detecting axillary lymph node metastases from breast cancer. *Eur J Cancer Clin Oncol*, **23**, 475–480.
141. Mazzeo, F., Accurso, A., Petrella, G. et al. (1986) Pre-operative axillary lymphoscintigraphy in breast cancer: experience with sub-areolar injection of 99Tcm-nanocolloidal albumin. *Nucl Med Commun*, **7**, 5–16.
142. Terui, S. and Yamamoto, H. (1989) New simplified lymphoscintigraphic technique in patients with breast cancer. *J Nucl Med*, **30**, 1198–1204.

143. Matsubara, S., Umehara, I., Shibuya, H. et al. (1986) Radionuclide lymphoscintigraphy performed on the mastectomized chest wall. *Cancer*, **58**, 1225–1230.
144. Saeki, T., Karaki, Y., Maeda, M. Honda, T. and Fujimaki, M. (1990) Development of Tc-99m labeled activated carbon microspheres and clinical application. *Nippon Geka Gakkai Zasshi*, **91**, 729–740.
145. Rossi, R. and Ferri, O. (1966) La visualizzazione della catena mammaria interna con Au-198. Presentazione di una nuova metodica: la linfoscintigrafia. *Minerva Med*, **57**, 1151–1155.
146. Schenck, P. (1966) Scintigraphische darstellung des parasternalen lymphsystems. *Strahlentherapie*, **130**, 504–508.
147. Ege, G.N. (1976) Internal mammary lymphoscintigraphy. *Radiology*, **118**, 101–107.
148. Matsuo, S. (1974) Studies of the metastasis of breast cancer to lymph nodes. II. Diagnosis of metastasis to internal mammary nodes using radiocolloid. *Acta Med Okayama*, **28**, 361–371.
149. Ege, G.N. (1977) Internal mammary lymphoscintigraphy in breast carcinoma: A study of 1072 patients. *Int J Radiat Oncol Biol Phys*, **2**, 755–761.
150. Bourgeois, P. and Fruhling, J.G. (1983) Internal mammary lymphoscintigraphy: current status in the treatment of breast cancer. *Crit Rev Oncol Hematol*, **1**, 21–47.
151. Dionne, L., Friede, J. and Blais, R. (1983) Internal mammary lymphoscintigraphy in breast carcinoma - a surgeon's perspective. *Semin Nucl Med*, **13**, 35–41.
152. Ege, G.N. and Elhakim, T. (1984) The relevance of internal mammary lymphoscintigraphy in the management of breast carcinoma. *J Clin Oncol*, **2**, 774–781.
153. Ege, G.N. and Clark, R.M. (1985) Internal mammary lymphoscintigraphy in the conservative management of breast carcinoma: an update and recommendations for a new TNM staging. *Clin Radiol*, **36**, 469–472.
154. Inga, G., Pepe, G., Caruso, M. et al. (1987) The detection of internal mammary lymph nodal chain metastases in breast cancer using radiolabelled colloids. *Eur J Gynaecol Oncol*, **8**, 105–109.
155. Van der Giessen, P.H. (1983) Parasternal lymphoscintigraphy as an aid in radiation treatment planning. *Strahlentherapie*, **159**, 422–426.
156. Collier, B.D., Palmer, D.W., Wilson, J.F. et al. (1983) Internal mammary lymphoscintigraphy in patients with breast cancer. Correlation with computed tomography and impact on radiation therapy planning. *Radiology*, **147**, 845–848.
157. Kaplan, W.D., Andersen, J.W., Siddon, R.L. et al. (1988) The three-dimensional localization of internal mammary lymph nodes by radionuclide lymphoscintigraphy. *J Nucl Med*, **29**, 473–478.

158. Hunt, M.A., Shank, B., McCormick, B. et al. (1989) The use of lymphoscintigraphy in treatment planning of primary breast cancer. *Int J Radiat Oncol Biol Phys*, **17**, 597–606.
159. Fisher, B., Ravdin, R.G., Ausman, R.K. et al. (1968) Surgical adjuvant chemotherapy in cancer of the breast: results of a decade of cooperative investigation. *Ann Surg*, **168**, 337–356.
160. Bonadonna, G., Valagussa, P., Moliterni, A., Zambetti, M. and Brambilla, C. (1995) Adjuvant cyclophosphamide, methotrexate, and fluorouracil in node-positive breast cancer. *N Engl J Med*, **332**, 901–906.
161. Handley, R.S. (1975) Carcinoma of the breast. *Ann R Coll Surg Eng*, **57**, 59–66.
162. Fisher, B., Redmond, C., Fisher, E.R. et al. (1985) Ten-year results of a randomized clinical trial comparing radical mastectomy and total mastectomy with or without radiation. *N Engl J Med*, **312**, 674–681.
163. Giuliano, A.E., Barth, A.M., Spivack, B., Beitsch, P.D. and Evans, S.W. (1996) Incidence and predictors of axillary metastasis in T1 carcinoma of the breast. *J Am Coll Surg*, **183**, 185–189.
164. Krag, D.N., Weaver, D.L., Alex, J.C. and Fairbank, J.T. (1993) Surgical resection and radiolocalization of the sentinel lymph node in breast cancer using a gamma probe. *Surg Oncol*, **2**, 335–340.
165. Giuliano, A.E., Kirgan, D.M., Guenther, J.M. and Morton, D.L. (1994) Lymphatic mapping and sentinel lymphadenectomy for breast cancer. *Ann Surg*, **220**, 391–401.
166. Uren, R.F., Howman-Giles, R.B., Thompson, J.F., et al. (1995) Mammary lymphoscintigraphy in breast cancer. *J Nucl Med*, **36**, 1775–1780.
167. Giuliano, A.E., Dale, P.S., Turner, R.R., Morton, D.L., Evans, S.W. and Krasne, D.L. (1995) Improved axillary staging of breast cancer with sentinel lymphadenectomy. *Ann Surg*, **222**, 394–401.
168. Springall, S.J., Rytina, E.R.C. and Millis, R.R. (1990) Incidence and significance of micrometastases in axillary lymph nodes detected by immunohistochemical techniques. *J Pathol*, **160**, 174.
169. Noguchi, S., Aihara, T., Motomura, K., et al. (1996) Detection of breast cancer micrometastases in axillary lymph nodes by means of reverse transcriptase-polymerase chain reaction. *Am J Pathol*, **2**, 649–656.
170. Uren, R.F., Howman-Giles, R.B. and Thompson, J.F. (1998) The value of pre-operative lymphoscintigraphy in breast cancer treatment. *Eur J Cancer*, **34**, 203–204.
171. Stibbe, E.P. (1918) The internal mammary lymphatic glands. *J Anat*, **52**, 257.
172. Grossman, F. (1896) *Ueber die axillaren lymphdrusen*. Berlin: Inaug Dissert C. Vogt.
173. Bobbio, P., Peracchia, G. and Pellegrino, F. (1962) Connessioni linfatiche presternali fra le regioni mammarie dei due lati. *Ateneo Parmense*, **33**, 95.

174. Rosen, P.P., Lesser, M.L., Kinne, D.W. and Beattie, E.J. (1983) Discontinuous or "skip" metastases in breast carcinoma. Analysis of 1228 axillary dissections. *Ann Surg*, **197**, 276–283.
175. Mornard, P. (1916) Etude anatomique des lymphatiques de la mammelle, au point de vue de l'extension lymphatique des cancers. *Rev Chir*, **51**, 462.
176. Gulec, S.A., Moffat, F.L., Carroll, R.G. et al. (1998) Sentinel lymph node localization in early breast cancer. *J Nucl Med*, **39**, 1388–1393.
177. Krag, D., Weaver, D., Ashikaga, T. et al. (1998) The sentinel node in breast cancer. A mulicenter validation study. *N Engl J Med*, **339**, 941–946.
178. Hortobagyi, G.N. (1998) Treatment of breast cancer. *N Engl J Med*, **339**, 974–984.
179. McMasters, K.M., Giuliano, A.E., Ross, M.I. et al. (1998) Sentinel-lymph-node biopsy for breast cancer - Not yet the standard of care. *N Engl J Med*, **339**, 990–995.

INDEX